FIT MAMA

• • •

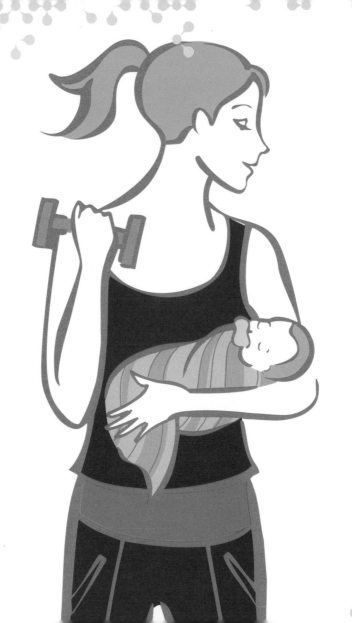

FIT MAMA

• • •

A Real-Life Fitness Guide for the New Mom

by Stacy Denney and Kate Hodson

Foreword by Susan Hollander, OB Nurse Practitioner
and Certified Nurse Midwife

Illustrations by Cindy Luu

CHRONICLE BOOKS
SAN FRANCISCO

Library of Congress Cataloging-in-Publication Data:

Denney, Stacy.

   Fit mama : a real-life fitness guide for the new mom / by Stacy Denney and Kate Hodson.

      p. cm.

   ISBN-13: 978-0-8118-5162-6

   ISBN-10: 0-8118-5162-1

1. Postnatal care. 2. Exercise for women. 3. Physical fitness for women.

I. Hodson, Kate. II. Title.

RG801.D39 2007

613.7'045–dc22

2006012071

Manufactured in China

Design by Amanda Poray

Distributed in Canada by Raincoast Books
9050 Shaughnessy Street
Vancouver, British Columbia V6P 6E5

10 9 8 7 6 5 4 3 2 1

Chronicle Books LLC
680 Second Street
San Francisco, California 94107
www.chroniclebooks.com

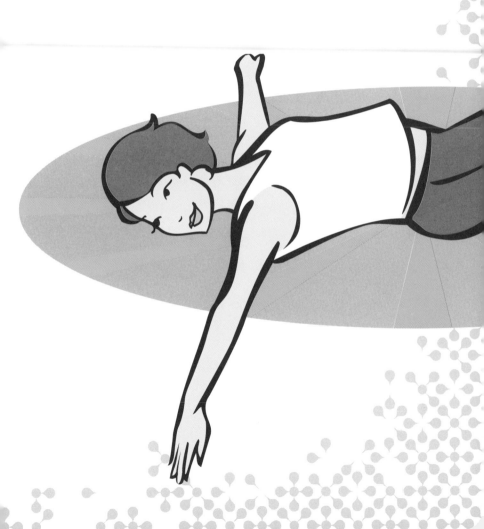

ACKNOWLEDGMENTS

• • •

Writing this book has been a long and sometimes exhausting journey. But thanks to the help and support of the following people, it's also been a thoroughly exciting one. We'd like to acknowledge their enormous contributions, without which we'd probably never have even taken the first step.

Jodi Davis of Chronicle Books, for the opportunity to make postpartum fitness seem like an attainable goal for more women than ever before (and to raise a smile or two in the process).

Susan Lawler, R.N., for her expertise and endless support, her love and amazing ability to give.

Justine Rudman, for introducing us to those wonderful yoga poses that allow us all to stay fit and connect with our children at the same time. We're constantly inspired by her determination to bring the benefits of yoga to as many new and expecting moms as possible.

DEDICATION

• • •

To Brad and Max, for their support and patience, and to all the new moms out there who have felt less-than-fit in those first postpartum months. Enjoy!
—SLD

To my husband, Luke, for his boundless enthusiasm and unfailing encouragement as this book took shape.
—KH

CONTENTS

• • •

FOREWORD

• • •

During the many years I've spent helping women have babies—and helping them adapt to their new roles after their babies have been born—it's been wonderful to see how the concept of prenatal exercise has gained credence within the medical population, and with expectant mothers themselves. Classes seem to have sprung up everywhere, bookstore shelves groan under the weight of the subject, and online communities spend hours discussing it.

However, it's always seemed to me that postpartum exercise is viewed as something of a poor relative. There are a handful of excellent books on the subject, but in reality, from a fitness perspective, the postpartum period is a field generally left unexplored and under-promoted. It's a shame because I'm certainly convinced of the benefits of postpartum exercise—the women I've seen who've exercised in the period following the birth of their babies just appeared more relaxed, and more physically able to cope with being a mother. They also seem happier with their bodies. And, as we all know, a happy mom means a happy baby.

For many women (even those who exercised consistently during their pregnancies), the notion of exercising after the birth of their babies is somehow unappealing. They're way too busy, way too tired, way too stressed—way too everything. This is terribly unfortunate, of course, as exercising regularly, and appropriately, in the weeks and months after the birth of a baby can have amazing effects on the mother, as well as facilitating her burgeoning relationships with her child and her child's other new parent.

That's why it's so gratifying to read *Fit Mama*, a book that actually stresses the importance of postpartum fitness while acknowledging the undeniable truth that the postpartum period can be grueling and disorienting, and often overwhelming. It also speaks to the fact that, in the real world, new moms don't have a lot of time or energy to plow through complicated routines and lengthy instructions, much less organize childcare and take three hours off to go to the gym every day.

I'm an advocate of *little and often* when it comes to postpartum exercise, of finding manageable exercises that are easy to do and that fit in around all the other things the new mother is doing. Motivation, of course, comes largely from within, but outside factors can help (or hinder). Above all, any exercise program should be enjoyable; at a minimum, that means an exercise routine should be straightforward, it shouldn't take hours to do, and there should be variety in terms of location (indoor and outdoor) and sociability (group or solo) to keep motivation going strong.

And it's most important to me, as a health care professional, that any fitness program endorses appropriate exercises—the right exercise at the right time. For the postpartum woman, it's critical that her chosen program spends time and focus on rebuilding the important muscle groups that are weakened during pregnancy and childbirth—the abdominals and pelvic floor—before moving on to aerobic exercises, cardio, yoga, and more.

Having been a postpartum woman myself, I know from personal experience that it's also a good idea to introduce some humor into the subject. The birth of a baby is an extraordinarily happy event, but one that has its fair share of tears. Most women experience predictable frustrations, worries, and concerns—about their babies, their parenting skills, and, pretty frequently, their changed bodies. And any book that puts these issues into perspective is definitely worth reading!

—Susan Hollander, OB Nurse Practitioner and Certified Nurse Midwife

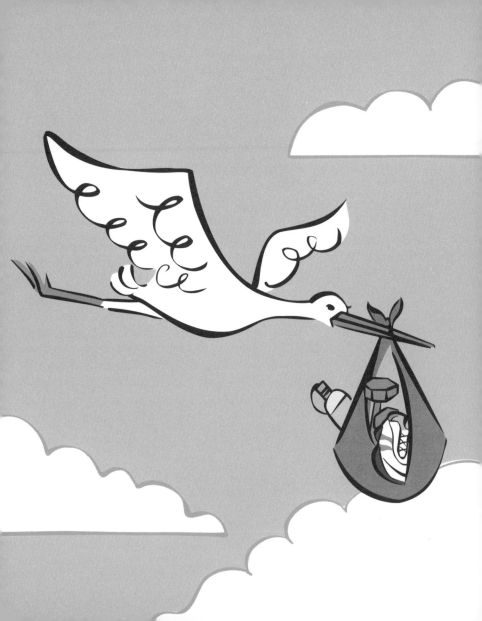

INTRODUCTION

•••

For many women, pregnancy is the easy bit. Although you may not realize it at the
time, there's a virtue in keeping all your mother/baby concerns neatly packaged in
one self-supporting unit (your belly). Sure, you feel nauseated, you develop hemorrhoids, and you find it hard to sleep, but assuming that you enjoy a fairly uneventful
and healthy pregnancy, your days are filled with nothing more troublesome than a
little ice cream–related heartburn or the discomfort you experience because your
arms are too short to stretch over your tummy to your computer's keyboard.

But then your baby arrives. And everything changes. Your lifestyle, your schedule,
your relationship with your partner, your body. Ah yes, your body. To be fair, your
body has been undergoing something of a transformation for the last nine months.
However, it's not until you give birth to your baby that the full extent of your
pregnancy-induced makeover will be revealed.

Right about now, we want to make the point that this is to be expected. Having a
baby is a huge physical deal. You can't expect to walk away looking like nothing much
happened. But, sadly, not everyone shares our belief. Society puts huge demands on
the new mom to stop looking like a new mom and start looking exactly like her old
self (fueled, no doubt, by those magazine photos of celebrity moms shaking their
pert little booties in their size 2 jeans just weeks after delivery). Sadly, and rather
bizarrely, it seems that the cult of the thin and the glamorous extends to new
mothers.

In our opinion, there's way too much pressure on the new mom to get back in shape
and simply not enough information about how to do it *and* stay healthy *and* adapt to
all the new stresses of motherhood. And that's why we wrote *Fit Mama*. It's the

happy collaboration of two fairly recently postpartum women, so you just know that we really, *really* understand exactly what you're going through. To convince you of our credentials on the subject, here's a little more about us and how this book came to be.

In September 2003, Stacy Denney opened Barefoot & Pregnant, a spa, fitness center, and resource center for pregnant women and new mothers in Marin County, Northern California. One year later she gave birth to a rather round baby, Max, after getting rather round herself (at least in the tummy area). As she came down from her postbirth high and the reality of her new body became all too apparent, she congratulated herself on cleverly surrounding herself with the kind of people who selflessly devote themselves to helping postpartum women get fit. But despite being in the business, so to speak, her return to fitness was no faster, and no easier, than any other new mother's.

During her pregnancy, Stacy had reconnected with Kate Hodson, an old friend who had just given birth to her second daughter, Molly. In days gone by, Stacy and Kate had bonded over Friday night exploits and several glasses of Chardonnay. But things were different now. By the time Stacy's Max was born, Kate was still feeling the effects of having a big baby more than six months before. It had, she realized, been easier the first time. After the birth of her first child in the summer of 2001, intensive breast-feeding and extensive walking had seen muscles tighten and weight shift relatively quickly. But a midwinter birth, coupled with a swifter return to a full-time job, put a dent in her plans the second time around. Help was required, and that's where Stacy—and her oh-so-useful Barefoot & Pregnant connections—came in.

United by a common belief in the importance of postpartum exercise—while acknowledging that some things are easier said than done—they pooled their knowledge, shared their experiences, and got writing. And the result is *Fit Mama*.

Whether you've just experienced a vaginal delivery or a cesarean birth, turn these pages for good advice about rebuilding your fitness level alongside simple exercises for your abdominal muscles, your pelvic floor, and your back, and chapters on stretching and strength training, cardio and classes, and more. But *Fit Mama* also deals with all the other factors in your life that contribute to your overall health and fitness—your new roles and responsibilities, your approach to nutrition, how well you sleep, your emotional health, where and when you connect with other moms, your relationship with your partner, and, of course, your baby.

That's because becoming a fit mama really isn't just about losing weight or getting back into shape. It's about appreciating the body that just did an unbelievable thing and being kind and considerate to the body that continues to do the most important job in the world—being a mother.

There is a school of thought (to which we subscribe) that says that once you've had a child and dealt with the sleeplessness and lack of personal space, the daily tears and hourly tantrums, you can pretty much do any job. We'd like to end with a similar analogy and remind you that if your body can create and grow and then deliver, on cue, *a whole other human being* (just think about it), then doing something as simple as losing a few pounds and tightening a muscle or two should be a breeze.

With that in mind, it's time to dust off your spandex, psych yourself up, and enjoy the journey to becoming a truly fit mama.

• • •

CHAPTER 1

BEFORE YOU START

Feeling good about getting fit

• • •

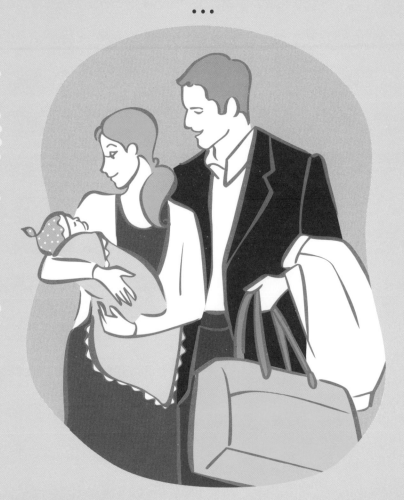

Perhaps you're reading this while your newborn snoozes on your chest. Perhaps you're being really proactive, and you're reading this even before your baby's been born. Either way, congratulations on becoming a mom, and congratulations on taking positive steps toward a fitter, healthier, and more energetic postpartum period.

Once you've relinquished the very appealing notion of putting your feet up with a large bowl of ice cream for the next several months, you'll come to realize that having a baby, and all that it entails, is the best motivation there is for getting fit. Along with satisfying a distinct preference for looking unpregnant now that your baby's in the world, postpartum fitness provides a multitude of additional benefits. Over the following pages, you'll learn why it's good for your physical health, your emotional well-being, and even the relationship you have with your new baby. You'll also learn about eating well, getting enough sleep (or at least trying to), and balancing the competing demands of your new life. And you'll learn that committing to a thoughtful, consistent exercise program almost as soon as you have your baby gives you the wonderful opportunity to be a fit mama for the rest of your life.

So this is it—your final opportunity to enjoy those last vestiges of what was hopefully an enjoyable and self-indulgent pregnancy. Make the most of it—lollygag your way through this chapter if you like—but know that sooner or later, the end will come. Or, rather, the beginning.

• • •

1. THE MISCONCEPTIONS OF MOTHERHOOD

Why they don't need to handle you with kid gloves

• • •

Pregnancy is not to be mistaken for a serious medical condition—multiple broken bones, for example—that requires you to do nothing but rest for weeks at a time. And while taking to your comfy, cozy bed for the last three or four months of your pregnancy, being waited on hand and foot, and generally living the life of the extremely pampered may sound like a fine idea, the reality is quite different. Just ask any woman who's spent any time on bed rest. Aside from the anxiety that comes with that particular situation, doing nothing gets boring after a while. There is, after all, only so much daytime TV the average constitution can tolerate. And it's nice to stretch your legs once in a while. However, a sedentary pregnancy was, in fact, the norm until quite recently.

A brief history of pregnancy and childbirth.
• • • • •

From the 1930s right up until the relatively hip and enlightened 1970s, pregnancy in the United States was thought of as a *delicate condition*, and those who suffered from it were expected to change their lives completely. In addition to the perceived risks (of which there were many, for both mother and child), pregnancy was also viewed as something of an irreversible state of affairs. The prevailing wisdom was that after being pregnant and having a baby, your body would never, *ever* be the same again. More specifically, your feet would grow a size, you'd lose a tooth, your breasts would sag, your hips would spread, and, most glamorous of all, every time you sneezed or coughed you'd pee your pants. Actually thinking about losing any extra weight you might have gained along the way? Don't even bother.

The really odd thing about this whole attitude toward pregnancy is that it had absolutely *no basis whatsoever* in scientific fact, mainly because nobody had ever actually bothered to get off their behinds and do some real research. It was, presumably, way more simple just to make it up, and over time such fallacies became medical fact. All of this meant that—in the absence of books on pregnancy, childbirth classes, and an Internet from which to access fascinating and instructive online quizzes—the average pregnant woman, pre-1970, was pretty much in the dark about the amazing thing that was happening to, and was about to emerge from, her own body.

Birthing a baby in those days was an entirely medical event, managed by (usually male) doctors, with little participation required from the woman—beyond doing the actual pushing—and certainly no input expected on the kind of birth she hoped to enjoy or (more likely) endure. Mind-numbing drugs were mandatory, and dads knew their place. Either they hovered outside in the corridor waiting to hand out cigars (if they were particularly involved in the process), or else they simply carried on with their lives while their womenfolk gave birth in isolation before being confined to a hospital bed, their newborns in the nursery, for a week or even two.

And if there was scant information on pregnancy and childbirth, there certainly wasn't *any* on the postpartum period, which, in any case, was less about how having a baby affected a woman's physical and emotional well-being and more about how swiftly she could incorporate her new role as a mother into her existing domestic routine. Then something changed.

Cue '70s disco music.
. . . . . .

Not for the first time, we have the feminist revolution to thank for a fundamental shift in thinking. On this particular occasion, it saved all manner of healthy women from unnecessarily boring and stifling pregnancies as they began taking real responsibility for their own bodies. The fitness revolution quickly followed, and women started wearing leg warmers and went jogging and got pregnant (though not necessarily as a direct result of each other). These pregnant fitness mavens soon found themselves on the horns of a dilemma—how to marry what they enjoyed about their new active lifestyles with the conventional wisdom about pregnancy. Such was the noise they created that a team of professionals was hastily gathered by the American College of Obstetrics and Gynecology and, as late as 1984, the very first guidelines for exercise during pregnancy were released.

Where we are today.
• • • • •

Since then, medical opinion has been changed and revised several times over. But the bottom line—now widely accepted and endorsed by medical data—is that a woman experiencing a normal pregnancy can have a better time of it, with fewer complications, and an easier transition into the postpartum period *if she exercises regularly*. And if exercise is good news for pregnant women, it's even better for new mothers. Think about it—your baby has been safely delivered, and now you can really focus on making your body your own again (well, as much as you can with a nursing infant attached to your chest). Yet, despite the wealth of evidence to support this fact, all sorts of myths and misconceptions continue to surround the subject of the postpartum period. Allow us the liberty of debunking a few of the more ridiculous.

Postpartum exercise: what's true and what's not.
• • • • • • • •

Myth: The softening hormones of pregnancy make you overly flexible and therefore more prone to joint injury.

Truth: While it's true that the group of hormones collectively called *relaxin* allow for the miraculous growth of a woman's body during pregnancy, a reversal of these effects occurs during the postpartum period. The best way to protect joints during pregnancy, the postpartum period, or at any time, for that matter, is to strengthen the muscles that move the joints. And the best way to do this is by exercising.

Myth: You shouldn't even think about exercising for the first six weeks after you give birth.

Truth: You can and should start exercising as soon as possible. Maybe you won't feel quite like stopping off at the gym on your way home from the hospital or birth center, but the sooner you make a start on gentle, restorative exercise to begin coaxing your abdominal and pelvic floor muscles back to their original supportive role, the better. Similarly, from the moment you hold your baby for the very first time, you should be mindful of proper posture. Your back will thank you in the long run.

Myth: You can't exercise while breast-feeding.

Truth: While having a baby clamped onto your left nipple may inhibit some degree of motion, breast-feeding as an activity is very compatible with exercise. Breast-feeding demands only a supportive bra, plenty of water, and enough extra calories to meet the demands of both an active lifestyle and milk production.

Myth: Your body will never be the same again.

Truth: Some of the physiological changes of pregnancy (like stretch marks, an expanded rib cage, and cesarean or episiotomy scars) are irreversible. But in terms of weight loss, muscular strength and tone, and overall endurance, it's possible to return to your old body. You may even find yourself with a better one.

2. HELP! SOMEBODY JUST GAVE ME A BABY

Finding your feet as a mom

• • •

You started your own babysitting business when you were thirteen. You have twenty-seven nieces and nephews. You've read every book ever written on newborn care. But as you hold your own baby in your arms, you realize that you have absolutely no idea what you are doing.

This small scrunched-up being is a complete and utter mystery to you. He makes funny faces, he cries for no apparent reason whatsoever, he poops and pees with no consideration for your soft furnishings, and he sleeps on a schedule (if you can call it that) that's the polar opposite of your own.

Being a mom is like no other job you've ever taken on. And, like no other, it's yours without any formal orientation. Babies don't come with an owner's manual, and there's no leaving early on a Friday afternoon either. While it's confusing and stressful, you are not without power in this situation. Here's what you can do to help yourself.

Take a baby honeymoon.

Designate the first four to six weeks after the birth of your baby as the initiation period into your new role and new lifestyle. This is the time you can and should take to get to know your baby, figure out his or her needs, figure out your own needs as a mom, and adjust to your new routine. And because it's a honeymoon (of sorts), it should be as relaxing and stress-free as you can possibly make it. This means no big projects, no entertaining hordes of people, and no commitments other than those that support you, your partner, and your baby.

Trust your intuition.
. . . .

This is one time to rely on your instincts. After all, women have been raising babies for millions of years and, for most of that time, without the benefit of hot and cold running water, disposable diapers, and parenting Web sites. Comfort yourself with the fact that babies are resilient little beings with demands that are actually pretty simple and, by and large, very easily met. They need food, they need to be warm and clean, and they need a modicum of entertainment. Most of all, babies need to be held and loved and comforted by you. If these needs are met, your baby will learn to trust that the world is a safe place—a place where he can feel relaxed and contented. And a relaxed and contented baby is usually accompanied by a mother of a similar disposition.

Make use of your resources.
. . . .

If you have questions, be sure to make good use of the ready-made army of experts around you—your parents, your friends, your pediatrician, the mothers in your moms' group, as well as your other resources—the books you read, the parenting classes you've taken, and the seemingly limitless information available online. Inevitably you'll encounter a whole range of different opinions, especially on certain more contentious topics like co-sleeping, vaccinations, and sleep training, but remember, only you know what's best for your own child. Just start believing it.

Take care of yourself.
. . . .

While your baby may seem to be the epicenter of your world, there is no more important person here than you. Your baby relies on you for everything she needs to survive, so you need to be physically and emotionally able to nurture her, physically and emotionally. Your first priority, therefore, is to take good care of your body and your mind. And that is where exercise comes in.

3. GETTING YOUR HEAD AROUND YOUR NEW BODY

Who'd have thought your boobs could actually get bigger?

• • •

Well, you have a new baby, and surprise, surprise, you have a new body, too. If you're more than a little shocked by the woman that you see in the mirror, reassure yourself that this is merely your *transitional* body, as, inside and out, the havoc wreaked on your person slowly but surely dissipates.

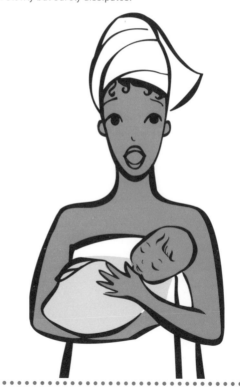

The good news is that you *will* get back in shape one day. For the vast majority of women, a beautiful, strong, healthy body is possible with a little desire, a little knowledge, and a little effort. In fact, depending on where you started from, you may even end up in better shape than before you got pregnant. But even if you were in amazing shape before you conceived, you probably won't ever return to your exact pre-pregnancy shape.

Many of the changes that occur during pregnancy reverse themselves within the first few weeks after the birth of your baby. Other pregnancy changes are more per-manent. Here's what you can expect to stay with you for life and what you can look forward to saying good-bye to.

The things that change.
• • • • • • •

Your tummy. Your abdominal muscles stretched and thinned throughout your pregnancy to allow for the growth of your baby, and they'll stay that way—weak and unsupportive—unless you take steps. These muscles are responsible for forward and lateral extension of the spine; they help keep your spine erect; and they're what you need if you want a flat(-ish) stomach. In short, these muscles are pretty darn useful, so you'll want them to be in good working order. Without them, you'll find yourself hunching forward as your body shifts its load to your less capable shoulders and upper and lower back. If you had a cesarean birth, you're probably even more *reluctant,* shall we say, to engage these muscles.

Your pelvic area. Your pelvic floor muscles are responsible for supporting your abdominal and pelvic organs against gravity. It comes as no surprise to learn, then, that they have an additional workload during pregnancy. Plus, they stretch significantly during a vaginal birth and may be additionally compromised if your perineum tears or you undergo an episiotomy. Like your abdominal muscles, they require gentle progressive exercise to return to their supportive state. The alterna-tive, should you still need convincing, is a future of potential urinary incontinence and painful sex.

Your uterus. Throughout the six weeks following the birth of your baby, your uterus works hard to shrink down to its pre-pregnancy size. This is accomplished by contractions (more noticeable in a second or subsequent delivery), accompanied by a vaginal discharge as your uterus sheds the lining that formed during your pregnancy. Known as *lochia,* this discharge starts off bright red in color before changing to brown and then a clearish yellow. While you may have a few other things on your plate right now, keep an eye on the color of the lochia. If, after changing from bright red to brown or yellow, it returns to a red color, take it as a sign that you are doing too much and that you should try to relax more.

Your weight. No matter how much weight you gained during your pregnancy, proper diet and exercise can help you return to a healthy weight. You'll shed the excess water weight in the first few weeks postpartum. Night sweats and, for that matter, day sweats are common. You'll also pee a lot and for a lot longer than you ever could later in your pregnancy, as your bladder can now hold more.

The things that may or may not change.

● ● ●

Your skin. While *chloasma,* or the mask of pregnancy—the result of an overproduction of melanin by the pituitary gland—often fades, it's still very important to wear sunscreen. The *linea negra*—the pigmented line that runs down the center of your abdomen—may or may not fade over time.

Your feet. During pregnancy, the hormone *relaxin* loosens the ligaments in your feet, causing the bones in your feet to spread, so it appears that your feet have grown a half size or so. They may or may not revert to their original size. If they don't, at least you have a great excuse to go shoe shopping.

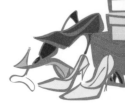

The things that you are likely stuck with.

• • •

Your rib cage. This expands during pregnancy and may never return to its original size. (The upside being that a larger rib cage creates the fortunate illusion that your waist is actually smaller than it is.)

Your breasts. If you are breast-feeding, your breasts will become, suddenly and quite amazingly, much heavier and fuller than ever before. Your fulsome pregnancy chest (which, just a few days ago, may have seemed quite impressive to you) pales by comparison. For all kinds of reasons, your new breasts might take some getting used to, as you and your infant occupy yourselves with the intricacies of breast-feeding. They may leak milk when you least expect it (your breasts, not your baby, although infants do this too). And, useful though they are, your new breasts may also exacerbate a tendency to hunch your shoulders. All of these changes may be noticeable for as long as you breast-feed, after which time your breasts will most likely be the same size and shape as they were before you got pregnant. If you decide to bottle-feed instead, your breasts will usually return to their normal size within a few weeks.

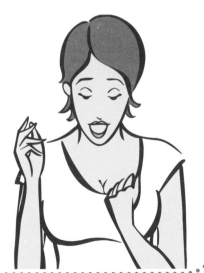

Your varicose veins. If you suffered from varicose veins during your pregnancy, know that while they will fade, they will always be there. The same goes for hemorrhoids (a type of varicose vein). They'll shrink but never disappear entirely. (Sorry about that.)

Your stretch marks. These will fade and eventually turn into silvery streaks.

Your cesarean scar. If you delivered your baby via cesarean, your abdominal or uterine scar will be with you for the long haul. The same goes for a perineal scar from an episiotomy or perineal tear.

The impact of these changes, temporary or otherwise, on your posture.
• • •
Over the last nine months, your whole abdominal and pelvic area slowly rearranged itself to accommodate your steadily growing baby. Quite suddenly, your baby is taking up space in the outside world. Now, your abdomen and pelvic area have the thankless task of returning your major organs to their original locations, something that usually takes about six weeks. You can't feel this happening, fortunately, although you may develop a not-so-attractive tendency to hunch forward—a tendency that is not helped by the new and frequent demands of your baby. Whether you are feeding your baby, changing his diaper, or lifting him into a bassinet or stroller, you will find yourself leaning over your child for what seems like hours every day. And while this is, of course, the best way to view your accomplishments and congratulate yourself on bringing such a splendid child into the world, your back will most definitely be less appreciative.

Remember, giving birth to a baby is a huge physical change that can have far-reaching consequences. While your body had nine whole months to get used to carrying your baby, childbirth gives it mere hours to adapt to your new, no-longer-pregnant state. Rest assured, however, that while you may not recognize the body you now have *(I still have a belly! My boobs are beyond big!)*, the changes you notice are to be expected. Best of all, they are mostly temporary. With proper diet and exercise, your body—internal organs, posture, and all—can return to one you know and love (or at least like) within several months.

4. GETTING YOUR HEAD AROUND YOUR NEW HEAD

And you thought you were hormonal before

• • •

You may have had a fantastic pregnancy, you may feel fully prepared to nurture your new baby, your house may be full of every device and article of clothing your progeny might need, but having a newborn in your life is a big change, and big changes take some getting used to. The psychological impact of, first, childbirth and, second, caring for a new baby can be huge. So, if your head is all of a whirl, there's probably a very good reason for it—or even seven.

You're disappointed in the birth experience.

Because of the quixotic nature of babies, very few birth experiences are exactly as planned, or expected, or even hoped for. If you had your heart set on an unmedicated birth and then had an epidural or a cesarean birth, you may feel swindled out of the kind of delivery day that you felt was rightfully yours.

You're adjusting to some powerful new hormones.

Your hormones have been in a state of flux for a long time. Now, things will start to change yet again as different hormones come into play. After the birth of your baby, there's a dramatic drop in your levels of estrogen, causing fatigue and mood swings (and maybe even vaginal dryness and thinning hair if you're really lucky).

You're getting less sleep.

• • • •

Especially with a first child, you will feel sleep-deprived. Incredibly so. Newborns need feeding at least every three hours, if not more often, and that's around the clock. If you're bottle-feeding, you may be able to share the night shift (or day shift) with a willing volunteer (i.e., your child's almost-as-exhausted other parent), but if you're breast-feeding—particularly in the early weeks and months—this is not always possible. Never underestimate the debilitating effect of sleep deprivation on your ability to function and on your ability to feel physically and emotionally in control of your immediate environment. Disturbed sleep patterns also tend to disrupt your daytime schedule, although, to be honest, the whole concept of schedule—as in being able to plan your day in order to successfully accomplish a number of tasks—is perhaps one you should dispense with fairly early on.

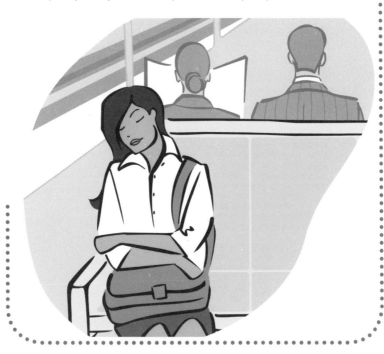

You lack confidence in your abilities.

• • •

If this is your first child, you will probably feel like you are setting out on uncharted territory with a small, squalling infant at the helm as your temperamental co-captain (and worse, one who's always hitting the bottle). As the journey progresses, your mounting uncertainty may become overwhelming. If, for example, you find breast-feeding difficult or your baby cries constantly, you may feel uncomfortable about leaving your home for anything more than a quick trip to the post office. This can be upsetting and demoralizing—after all, you think to yourself, you're a capable and efficient woman and you can't even manage a little tiny baby.

Your relationship with your partner shifts.

• • • •

No longer an intimate, exclusive twosome, your relationship now comprises three people—you, your partner, and the person that's attached to your side 24/7. The net result? *You* may miss the alone time with your partner and at the same time feel resentful that the burden of parenting in these early days falls mainly on your shoulders. *Your partner* may feel excluded from the cozy relationship you're establishing with your new baby and neglected by you (because, clearly, you are rather busy attending to someone else). Either way, harsh words may be spoken, feelings may be hurt, and tantrums (thrown by either one of you) may take place.

You're forced to relinquish control.

• • • •

Before you had your baby, you most likely had a job with responsibilities. You definitely had day-to-day contact with other, usually rational, adults. You put gas in your car, maintained a balance in your bank account, bought unsuitable shoes, and enjoyed happy hour on a regular basis. In short, You Were In Charge. Being a mother is about relinquishing control over your time, over your social life, even over your ability to enjoy a quiet moment with your brand-new copy of *People* magazine, and this can be hard to accept. These days, it seems like it's all about your baby's schedule and your baby's needs. It seems like this because it is like this.

You feel your old friends can't relate to your new situation.
• • •

In the good old days, you and your pals connected over the lives and loves of your favorite celebs, exploits from your college years, or a shared appreciation of fine wine. Now it feels like you have nothing in common with your babyless friends. They go to work, plan vacations, and get their nails done; you feed your baby around the clock, watch daytime soaps, and feel saddened by the fact that you're losing touch with your buddies.

Any of the above can bring on mild postpartum depression, also known as the *baby blues*. And while it's not uncommon to feel sad, tearful, unmotivated, and lethargic in the early postpartum period, it's not something you should take lightly or accept as par for the course. Feeling low doesn't have to be something that comes automatically with the big boobs and the perpetual smear of spit-up on your shoulder. If you believe that you're suffering from mild postpartum depression, try to take the following steps.

Reconnect with your partner.
• • • • • • •

Spend at least five minutes a day talking to your partner about anything but the baby. Your joint production may be the hottest topic around, but your relationship will benefit if you engage each other on other subjects and on other levels.

Ask for help.
• • •

And be direct about it. Tell your family and your friends that if they want to see your new baby, they have to bring a meal, pick up groceries, or do a load of laundry.

Treat yourself.
• • • •

Get a massage, a manicure, or a facial while your partner looks after the baby. Everybody will benefit from the two or three hours you spend in the spa. You'll feel more relaxed, and your partner will get to work on important parenting skills.

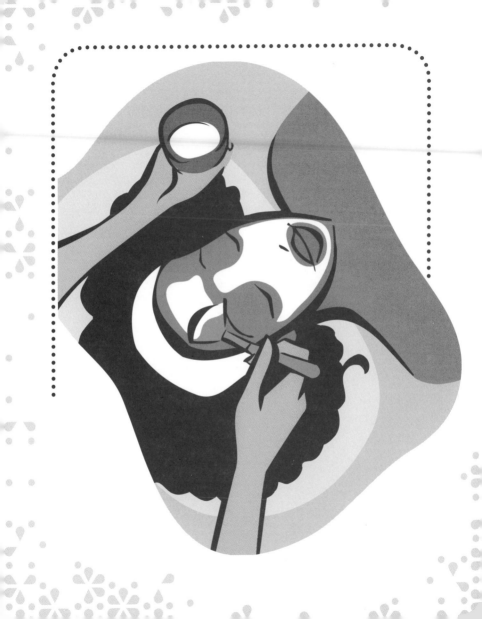

Develop a baby-centric social circle.
· · · · ·

If your friends don't have babies, consider seeking out women who are going through the same experience as you. Call somebody from your childbirth preparation class or join a mothers' group. More than any other activity, connecting with other new moms will help banish those feelings of isolation.

Learn how to lift your own spirits.
· · · ·

Have a ready-made strategy or two up your sleeve for when things get to be too much. Identify what can make you feel better—maybe it's picking up the phone to call your mom or putting the baby in the stroller and getting outside in the fresh air— and do it.

It's important that you recognize when you start to feel overwhelmed, as this may be a sign that your baby blues are developing into moderate or severe postpartum depression, conditions that require medical attention. Be on the lookout for telltale signs like inertia, sadness, lethargy, and weepiness. If you are experiencing deep feelings of depression that persist, are unable to care for yourself or your baby, have irrational thoughts, or hear voices, you must seek help from your health care professional immediately.

5. WHY IT'S PHAT TO BE FIT

The very real benefits of postpartum exercise

• • •

If you were smart enough to exercise during your pregnancy, then you have three things to look forward to in the postpartum period. Your body will feel better (i.e., less traumatized by long hours of labor and childbirth). You will probably look better than you might expect (which will give you a big psychological boost). And you'll be better prepared to take on the very physical tasks of motherhood.

If, however, the idea of exercising kind of slipped your mind for forty or so weeks, all is not lost. Just remember that the sooner you start after the birth of your baby, the sooner you'll start to feel better on all counts. And whichever camp you *honestly* fall into, know that the benefits of a regular postpartum exercise routine are huge.

The physical advantages of postpartum exercise.
• • •

Your postpartum recovery will be smoother. Whether you gave birth vaginally or via cesarean, exercise can make you feel better, faster. It can help return your internal organs to their pre-pregnancy arrangement (per your high school biology textbook), and reassuringly, it'll give you more control over those areas that grew so dramatically during your pregnancy. Even, you'll be thrilled to hear, your hemorrhoids.

You'll grow stronger. Being a mother is a physically demanding job. Even though you're no longer pregnant, you'll still find yourself carrying your baby for hours at a time. Plus, as every room in your house confirms, babies come with a lot of equipment. When you're hefting your baby plus the car seat, the diaper bag, and the stroller, you'll be very glad that your body is up to it.

You'll have more energy. Exercising gives you more energy, which, as a mother, you'll find more than useful. All right, so your baby is fairly stationary right now. But that relaxing state of affairs won't last forever. Pretty soon he'll be a two-year-old wreaking havoc at the mall. Right about then you'll be glad you can keep up with him.

You'll become generally healthier. Exercise, postpartum or otherwise, increases your metabolism. It lowers your blood pressure, pulse, and respiratory rate and makes for a healthier respiratory and cardiovascular system. Do it on a regular basis, and you'll increase your body's muscular strength, become more flexible, and boost your endurance. And (the really good news) you'll be able to burn fat stores more efficiently.

But your body isn't the only thing that benefits from postpartum exercise. Regular exercise can have significant and powerful effects on your mental health too. It can increase your energy levels, as we've said before, and perhaps more important, it can reduce susceptibility to postpartum depression. Here's why committing to a postpartum exercise program is especially good for your head.

The mental benefits of postpartum exercise.
● ● ●

You'll find yourself connecting with other new moms. Sure, you can make your exercise routine a solitary venture. But join a formal exercise class for new moms or create your own informal exercise group with a few friends from your childbirth class, and you've got yourself a ready-made support group. You'll bond over the traumas of unsympathetic partners, lack of sleep, and the exorbitant cost of maxi pads. Just talking with other women who are going through what you're going through (albeit with a *much* less attractive baby in tow) can be hugely reassuring.

You'll feel better about your physical appearance. There's no denying it—how your body looks affects how you feel about yourself. Exercise can help you take control over your body and make it easier to lose your pregnancy weight,

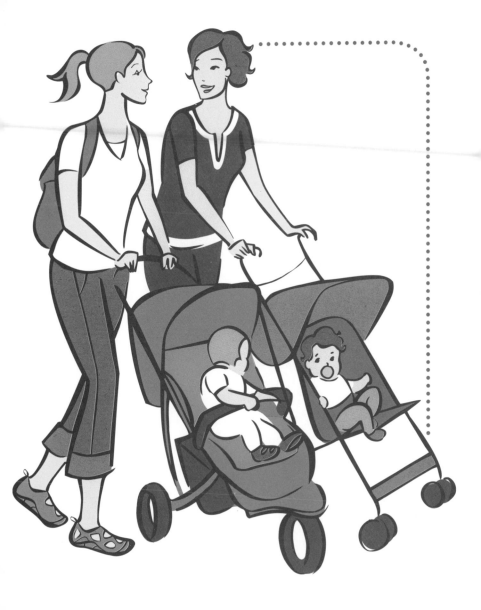

increase your muscle tone, and gain a flatter stomach. And you'll probably feel better just *knowing* that it can also help reduce your risk of incontinence in later life.

You'll boost your metabolism. A regular and consistent exercise program increases your metabolic rate, which helps you burn fat faster. Getting in shape can be hugely motivating, and seeing real results can give you a more positive outlook on your new baby-centered way of life.

You'll increase your level of endorphin production. Your body produces these "natural opiates" as a response to activity. Still hardwired for primeval woman, your brain thinks that when you expend energy you are fleeing from a saber-toothed tiger or similarly prehistoric threat, when you're really attempting to get away from the extra pound or two currently residing on your butt. These feel-good hormones make you feel calmer, happier, and less receptive to pain (so, of course, you'll be game for another circuit before heading home).

Whichever way you look at it, you'll reap the benefits of regular postpartum exercise for years to come. Embark on a program now, and you'll still be enjoying its positive effects when *your baby* is having *her own babies*.

6. EATING FOR TWO, AGAIN

New-mom nutrition for your new-mom lifestyle

• • •

You're delighted with your new baby but less so with your new body. This is not, however, the time to go on a diet. In any case, you don't really need to. Know that having lost ten pounds or so at delivery, you will lose a further ten in the first two weeks of your baby's life. After that, your overall weight loss will vary, depending on how much weight you gained during your pregnancy and how you approach your postpartum life.

As you transition into this next phase, nothing is more important than what you put into your body, especially if you are breast-feeding. Follow these basic guidelines, and you'll develop eating habits that will support your new way of life, as well as providing the foundation for weight loss in the long run.

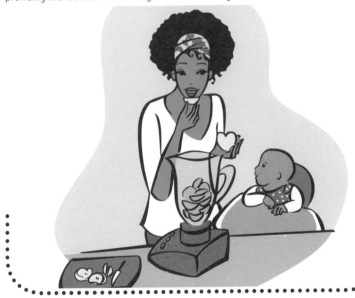

Drink, drink, drink.

Water it is. This is very important during the first few days after you give birth when you may be swollen, especially if you received IV fluids during your labor. At this time, you may also be losing an above-average amount of fluid. Night sweats are normal right now, as is peeing a lot as your body releases excess fluids stored during pregnancy. Along with avoiding dehydration, water also helps to keep constipation and hemorrhoids at bay, as well as maintaining your breast milk supply. Drink at least one eight-ounce glass of water every time you breast-feed.

Keep taking your prenatal vitamins.

If you took them during your pregnancy, don't stop now. Many formulations are created specially to support both pregnant and lactating women, and even if you are not breast-feeding, your eating habits may be less than stellar as you adjust to your busy new lifestyle.

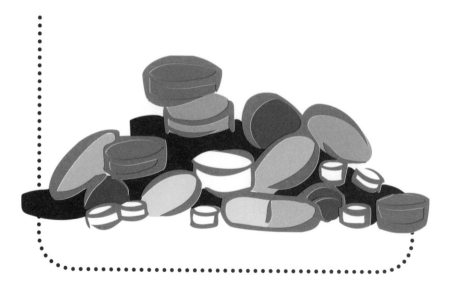

Eat small and often throughout the day.

Chances are you're not going to be whipping up a gourmet dinner every evening. However, you do need to refuel often, so make sure you have plenty of healthful comestibles at hand. During the early postpartum period, you should try to consume the equivalent of your pregnancy diet plus an extra 200 or so calories. (If you're not breast-feeding, just eliminate those additional calories.)

Stock up on healthful snacks.

By some strange twist of fate, it seems to be that high-sugar, high-fat snacks are the only things you can lay your hungry little hands on when you're refilling your water bottle after your baby's lengthy 3:00 A.M. feed. Avoid temptation by stocking the fridge, the pantry, and, indeed, any available counter space with nutritious and healthful snacks that require minimal preparation. Things like cheese, fruit, rice cakes, yogurt, and celery loaded with peanut butter are easy ways to give your body energy and satisfy cravings.

Think about breast-feeding.

As well as being a wise choice for your child, anecdotal evidence suggests that breast-feeding can help you lose weight. There's no medical data to prove this, and it doesn't work for every woman, but there's way more good than harm to be had in trying.

7. BUT I'M TOO EXHAUSTED TO EXERCISE

How to do less and sleep more

• • •

While being a new mom means you've gained so many wonderful new things—
a baby, a house full of complicated equipment, the ability to get all teary-eyed over
small undergarments—there are quite a few things it appears you have lost. These
include the ability to secure a good night's sleep on a regular basis, the ability to get
anything other than baby-focused tasks accomplished, and the ability to dredge up
enough energy to shower and dress in the morning without feeling like you have to
go lie down for an hour or two.

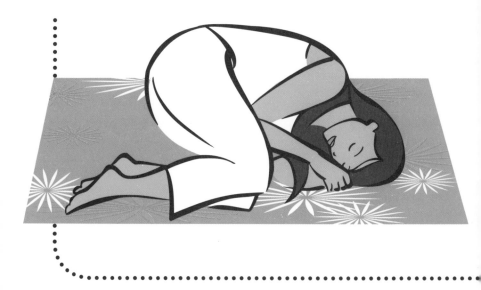

Issue #1: *The lack of sleep.*
· · · · · ·

While adapting to life with a baby can be anything from a little bit overwhelming to completely traumatic, it's primarily exhausting (in an overwhelming and/or traumatic way). The degree of exhaustion you will experience is contingent on several factors. Assuming that you had a normal and safe delivery and that your newborn is healthy, it depends on his temperament (some babies are naturally placid, others seem to make a career choice out of hollering), how well the feeding is going (easily for both of you, a long and painful struggle, or somewhere in between), and the environment you come home to (ideally a freezer full of meals, helpful friends on tap, and a loving partner just waiting to satisfy your every whim).

However, it's important to note that these factors determine not *whether* you will be tired, but *how* tired you will be (on a scale of one to ten, where "one" is "perpetually yawning" and "ten" is "nonfunctioning zombie"). Babies, mellow or otherwise, need feeding 'round the clock, so your sleep patterns cannot help but be disturbed. Babies also like to be held constantly, which makes doing any other vaguely useful life-supporting task (like taking a shower or fixing breakfast) virtually impossible. That means that when your baby sleeps, you'll find yourself catching up on domestic tasks and matters of personal hygiene as opposed to doing the most necessary thing of all—sleeping.

Since tiredness is a given during the early postpartum period, the idea of actually having the energy (not to mention the inclination) to exercise may seem so ridiculous as to make you laugh. Or cry. Please don't do either. Instead, focus on reprioritizing your daily tasks, and identify those that can bubble away quite happily on the proverbial back burner.

For example, a baby certainly seems to increase your "to do" list exponentially, but only if you consider things like doing a load of laundry a day or writing ten thank-you cards an hour *must-dos*. The only thing that is an absolute must-do right now is *taking good care of yourself*. And a big part of that is getting enough sleep.

In fact, anything that helps you stay healthy, happy, and sane during these weeks and months is an absolute priority—which is why you should also think about including exercise in your new list of must-dos. Exercise increases your energy levels and helps you sleep better (thus maximizing the benefit of the precious few hours of night-night that you do get). And while the prospect of working up a sweat (when you could be happily lying in the fetal position on your newborn's bedroom floor) probably feels untenable, know that there is a wealth of medical data to back up this fact. Honestly.

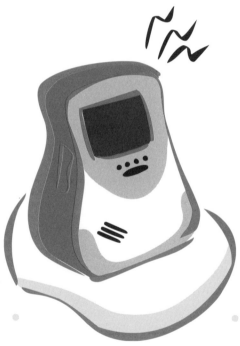

At the very least, make a commitment to walk for five minutes every day. You can do this with your baby (extra points for pushing a stroller) or by yourself while your partner looks after your progeny. It's even easier if you hook up with a friend from your childbirth class or mothers' group. After only a few days, you'll probably start to feel your energy level quiver a little, maybe even rise a nano-notch or two. Seize on these positive feelings, and increase your walk time to ten or, if you're feeling particularly adventurous, fifteen minutes a day.

Issue #2: *The lack of productivity.*

Before your baby entered the world, it was relatively easy to be organized. You'd set an hourly goal or three (finish writing that report, check online for the current relationship status of the Hollywood couple du jour, call your best friend), you'd make a mental (or, for safety's sake, an actual) "to do" list, and then you'd launch yourself into action. Spell-check that document! Log on to celebritytrash.com! Hit speed-dial!

Multitasking was the norm. You were good at it, and heck, you liked projecting the confident aura of a busy professional woman hacking her way through the problems (sorry, *challenges*) of the day. But things have changed. In many ways, having a baby slows the pace down. Way, way down. And even if you'd like to move a little faster, there's really no choice but to fit in with your baby's preferred way of doing things. After all, we all know who's going to complain (loudly) should you foolishly decide to rush through a feed or skip a diaper change.

If you're coming to this mom thing straight from a fairly fast-paced lifestyle, failure to achieve even the simplest endeavor can leave you feeling frustrated. You can't help but think, *if I can't even find the time to stock up on bottled water and a couple of gallons of ice cream, how in the world am I going to find the time to exercise?* The answer is to draw on the time-saving skills you used in your pre-baby life.

Multitask. Pre-baby, your multitasking might have been all about filing your nails while on speakerphone or whipping up a casserole while reading the newspaper. As a new mom, you'll find that there are many tasks that not only incorporate exercise but make expending energy completely unavoidable. At the lower end of the *Gosh, that sounds like fun* spectrum are activities like cleaning house and gardening, which you can do with your baby supervising from her car seat or bouncy chair. Some activities actually require the willing participation of a baby volunteer, such as pushing a stroller (hang a heavy diaper bag on the handles and you can call it weight training), taking a mom-and-baby yoga class, and breast-feeding, which, while not strictly an exercise, is an activity that consumes an extra 500 or so calories a day.

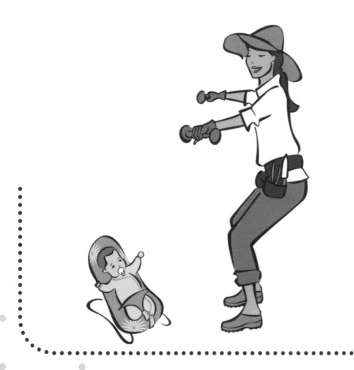

Delegate. If finances allow, consider hiring a cleaner, ordering your groceries online and having them delivered to you, and taking your laundry to the wash-and-fold place. Granted, these services aren't free, but they'll buy you some much-needed extra time that, over the course of a week, you can use for *you time* (that you can spend exercising, of course). If you'd rather not spend the money, delegate everyday tasks to people who won't charge you (i.e., your friends and relatives). Cash in all those offers to come and help out, and don't feel bad. It's to everybody's advantage that you pay attention to your mental health.

Issue #3: *The lack of energy.*
• • • • • •

Here's the plan. You sort out Issue #1 (lack of sleep) by spending less time on the unimportant stuff. You sort out Issue #2 (lack of productivity) by delegating the tasks that are necessary. And hey presto, no more Issue #3 (lack of energy). Sound easy? We know it's not. But at least it's a game plan, and it might provide you with a little clarity as you attempt to come to terms with your confusing and disorienting new way of life.

The bottom line is, do less, sleep more, make time to exercise, and you'll find looking after your baby easier and less stressful. Remember, you come first. Don't confuse motherhood with martyrdom (a common mistake). Start to do that as soon as your baby is born, and you can fast-forward a dozen years to the day that you volunteer to drive all the neighborhood kids to soccer practice while their own mothers get pedicures. It's not a pretty sight.

8. SPANDEX? CHECK!
STATIONARY BICYCLE? CHECK!
BOUNDLESS ENERGY? ER . . .

Find out if you're ready to get fit

• • •

Different women come around to the notion of postpartum exercise at different times. Sure, intellectually, you know that it's a good idea, but putting theory into practice isn't always easy. But whether you're incredibly committed (or else still high on a not-unpleasant cocktail of birthing narcotics) and start exercising the day after you deliver your baby or you give yourself a month (or six) before you even start to think it might be a good idea makes no difference—everybody pretty much starts from the same point and with the same kind of exercises. Sooner is better, of course, but if you start later, you still have to start at the beginning. Remember, your goal is not to instantly get back into your belly-baring jeans but to coax your pelvic and abdominal muscles back to their original supportive roles as you focus on proper posture for your new body.

The exercises that can help you achieve these goals don't require a lot of energy, but they do require commitment. Later on, you can look ahead to increasing the frequency, duration, and intensity of your workout, but before you do anything, make sure you're physically ready to start exercising. Take this little self-test (and no cheating).

How fit were you before you became pregnant? If you were the original couch potato, having a baby is not going to change your basic level of fitness, and you should start slowly. Very, very slowly. If you were fit before, your level now may be intermediate rather than beginner, but you'd be smart to focus on your form rather than on speed and intensity. Remember, the body you're working out with now is not the one that you're used to.

SCORE YOURSELF:

3 points   I used to run marathons.

2 points   I had a gym membership.

1 point   What's a gym?

Did you exercise during your pregnancy? If you didn't exercise at all, start out slowly. Even if you did exercise, you may be surprised at how quickly and easily you get fatigued these days. Take this into consideration when planning your exercise routine.

SCORE YOURSELF:

3 points   I went through three pairs of running shoes.

2 points   I walked ten blocks daily just to get to the gelato store.

1 point   I just couldn't seem to find maternity jogging shorts.

What kind of pregnancy did you have? If you had complications that put you on bed rest, you should talk to your doctor or midwife before embarking on an exercise program.

SCORE YOURSELF:

3 points   I never felt better. Seriously, I can't wait to do it again.

2 points   I was tired and cranky. I still am.

1 point   I lay in bed for twenty-four long, long weeks.

What kind of birth did you have? Having a cesarean birth, an episiotomy, or suffering from excess blood loss may mean that you are still more fatigued than you might realize. Again, you should start any exercise program slowly and talk to your doctor or midwife first.

SCORE YOURSELF:

3 points   It was like shelling peas.

2 points   It was everything they said it would be, only longer and more painful.

1 point   Anesthesia and sutures were involved.

NOW, CALCULATE YOUR FITNESS READINESS QUOTIENT.

4-6 points   *Take it easy.* Don't push yourself too hard—you've got plenty of time.

7-9 points   *Off you go.* It sounds like you're ready to get moving.

10-12 points   *You've already gone.* See you later!

Your score reveals only how fast (or how slow) you can expect to progress. Regardless of your current or former fitness level, your starting point—mastering the basics—is the same as everybody else's. Which means that it's now time to move on—at a suitably brisk pace—to the next chapter.

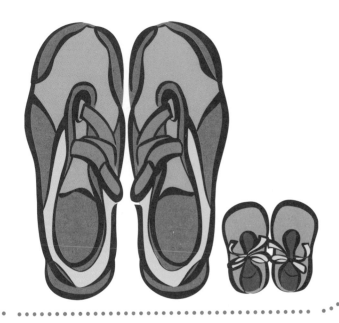

CHAPTER 2

THE FIRST WEEK

It's never too soon to get fit (honestly)

...

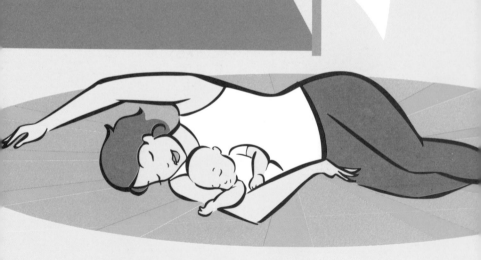

Well, you've written all your thank-you cards, done several loads of laundry, bathed the baby (twice), scrubbed the spit-up out of the carpet, and now there's no avoiding it: it's time to exercise. First of all, kudos for getting this far. It says you're committed to the idea, at least, of getting fit, and that's half the battle. And because this is your first week of postpartum exercise, which may or may not be the first week after your baby's birth, we'll be easy on you.

Your body's been through a lot. It's overworked and exhausted, it's been stretched and pulled, and quite frankly, it needs more than a little encouragement if you want to even *start* to reverse the effects of the previous forty (plus) weeks. But this is not the time to begin training for a triathlon. Speed and endurance are not, you'll be relieved to hear, part of your new exercise vocabulary. Instead, familiarize yourself with two key—and low-key—concepts: *awareness* (of your body and how it moves) and *consistency* (with regard to a safe and gentle exercise routine).

To that end, this chapter focuses on the basics—a collection of pretty simple exercises that are vital to master before you move on to other things. At this stage it's all about strengthening your abdominals, making your pelvic floor muscles more supportive, and realigning your spine. Pretty soon, we'll have you breathing from your diaphragm, contracting your Kegels, and tilting your pelvis.

If it all sounds horribly active, don't worry. Most of these exercises take the form of small and subtle movements that you can do in a comfortably horizontal position. But what you do here and now forms the very foundation of all the exercises that follow and, indeed, any type of exercise you do, from weight training, swimming, and yoga to stroller pushing, baby lifting, and car seat installing. Spend some quality time here, and you'll soon be on the road to postpartum fitness.

1. WHO KNEW MOTHERHOOD WAS SUCH A WORKOUT?

What they don't tell you about babies

• • •

Sickening, isn't it, when you think of all those years you dragged your reluctant body to the gym at some ungodly hour of the morning or took yourself on an early evening run while all your friends were enjoying happy hour, and all you had to do to get your daily workout was look after a teeny-weeny baby. Here's how you'll be getting fit from now on.

Unexpected weight training sessions.

A seven-and-a-half-pound newborn weighs about the same as your capacious everyday handbag, the one that's packed with a cosmetic purse, a selection of reading material, and your day planner (basically all the things you won't be needing for a while). It's not, at first glance, a particularly hefty weight. You have no problem carrying it to and from work and on shopping expeditions. But the difference between your seven-and-a-half-pound baby and your seven-and-a-half-pound bag is that you can put your bag under a chair and leave it there for hours at a stretch and you won't hear a whimper.

Babies, on the other hand, like to be held *constantly* (in your arms, over your shoulder, in a sling, or in a baby-carrier). They like to snuggle as close as they possibly can. It's more convenient for feeding for one thing, and it generally makes them feel more secure. But from your point of view, it's like a never-ending weight training session. And you can add to this the fact that your baby's bulk is on an upward trajectory, as he gains anything from a few ounces a week to more than a pound. (Handbags don't typically do this, either.)

Unanticipated aerobic workouts.
• • • • • • • • • •

Your life, pre-baby, might have found you being somewhat sedentary—sitting at a desk, sitting on public transport, sitting in a local coffee emporium, or sitting in front of your TV. Sure, your days may have required you to trot from point A to point B and back again. And, yes (for argument's sake), you were sensible and maintained a moderate pregnancy exercise regime that included walking and swimming. But being a mom calls for rigorous and sustained daily—nay, hourly—activity as you lift your baby from the crib to your knee, into the stroller, onto the changing table, onto your shoulder, and back into the bassinet. And then you're constantly bending over to pick up discarded toys, or to push the stroller, or to lift heavy equipment—like that foolishly overpacked diaper bag—in and out of your car.

But hefting a baby around is not just about supporting a weight. Your baby probably requires that you move around at a very specific pace and with a very exact rhythm while you hold him. This may be something of a shock to your system (not to mention your body). All this lifting and bending and pushing and carrying and walking is really and truly a great workout, as long as your body is in tip-top shape. If it's not—and right now, to be perfectly honest, it's probably not—all these exhausting new activities will only compound the stress and strain your body is under following the birth of your baby. It's just one more reason to turn the page and get started on the real exercises (or at least the ones you can do while lying down).

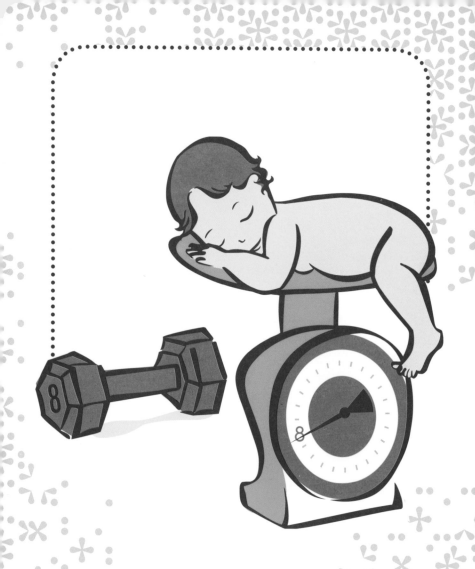

2. LOVING THAT POSTBABY BELLY

What happens to your tummy after delivery

• • •

Who'd have thought you'd be proud of having a large tummy? But there's nothing quite like that tight-as-a-drum belly stretched over a pretty much full-term baby to inspire delight in yourself and horrified fascination in others. It's a shame, then, that the same cannot be said for your belly just a week or so later. Yes, it's still big. Yes, you still look pregnant. But now it's about as taut as a water bed. And despite having a new and demanding baby to take your mind off things, you may be wondering where on earth your new-style tummy came from and, more to the point, what the chances are that you can return it and get your money back.

Let's start with the easy bit—the whys and wherefores (as opposed to the what-to-dos) of your postpartum belly.

Problem child #1: *Your stretched abdominal muscles.*

During pregnancy, as you know, your uterus expanded massively. Really massively. Your abdominal muscles—presumably reluctant to miss out on a change of scenery—came along for the ride and stretched themselves out over your big old belly for the whole nine-month pleasure trip. The bad news (not that you haven't already noticed this yourself) is that these muscles don't immediately ping back into shape just as soon as your baby squeezes himself out. You can also blame the excess fat and fluid your body stored during pregnancy and in anticipation of any breast-feeding that you might be doing for your current fulsomeness. And if you had a cesarean birth, you may also have additional swelling to compound the issue.

But your new belly is not just a cosmetic I'll-never-be-able-to-wear-a-bikini-again kind of a situation. As well as contributing to that still-pregnant appearance, your weakened abdominals may also indirectly (via a misaligned pelvis and by way of an unsupported lumbar region) be causing backache.

Yet, the good news is that deep down, however compromised, you are still the proud owner of four sets of major abdominal muscles, all with the potential to return to their former bounce-a-quarter-on-'em look and feel. Fighting fit or not, they're layered like a lasagna, one set on the left-hand side of your body and one on the right. The deepest layer is the *large transverse abdominus*. On top of them, along the midline of your abdomen, are the *recti* muscles. On top of them are the *internal obliques*. And on top of them are the *external obliques*.

Working in different combinations, these four sets of muscles move and stabilize the upper part of your torso. And working all together, they help you breathe. This means that the best (i.e., the easiest and most efficient) way to work *all* your abdominals *all at once* is by making correct *abdominal breathing* part of your every-day—well, every minute, really—life.

Also known as *diaphragmatic breathing*, abdominal breathing is a surprisingly effective way of encouraging your abdominal (and pelvic) muscles to return from whence they came. It can also help your postpartum body shake off the effects of birthing medication and anesthesia. And it's pretty relaxing, as your frequent practice of the following exercise will prove.

EXERCISE: ABDOMINAL BREATHING

Frequency: Ten times a day

When you're comfortable doing this exercise lying down, try it while sitting or standing.

1   Lie down on the floor or bed. With your knees bent and comfortably apart, allow the weight of your upper torso to sink into the surface you're lying upon.

2   Gently place your hands on your belly, and close your eyes.

3   Inhale, and concentrate on sending the breath to your abdominal area, as if you were trying to inflate a balloon inside your belly. As your abdominal muscles relax and your lungs expand fully, your hands will rise.

4   Exhale, and imagine that you're deflating the balloon by pushing all the air outside your body. Allow your abdominal muscles to contract as your hands sink into your belly.

Problem child #2: *Your separated recti muscles.*
• • • • • • • • • • • • •

The thick layer of Jell-O currently cocooning your once-firm belly may not be the only novelty you've noticed between your boobs and your hips. Perhaps you're one of the new moms who suffer from *diastasis recti*, the visible separation between your left and right recti muscles. Caused (once again) by the circulating hormones of pregnancy, this condition requires that you modify any exercise program in order to avoid further separation of the muscles.

Not sure if you have diastasis recti? Here's a handy little self-exam: Lie on your back, with your knees bent and your chin tucked in. Then slowly raise your head over your shoulders, with your arms stretched out in front of you. If you're a diastasis recti kind of gal, you'll see a somewhat alarming bulge in the middle of your abdominal area. You may be able to insert (even more alarmingly) several fingers horizontally into the soft region between your separated muscles. It's reason enough to spend some time on the following exercise.

EXERCISE: THE STITCH-UP

Frequency: Ten times a day

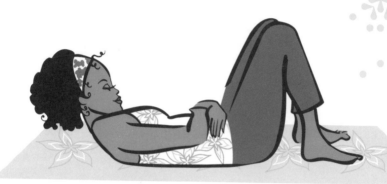

Try doing this before getting out of bed in the morning, when you're lying in bed just before you go to sleep at night, or when you find yourself in a horizontal position on a level surface (perhaps upon waking from that spontaneous nap on the living room floor).

1   Lie on your back with your knees bent.

2   Cross your hands over your abdomen so that your right hand is on your left recti muscle and your left hand on the right recti muscle.

3   With your shoulders flat on the floor, raise your head while slowly exhaling.

4   As you bring your head forward to your chest until you're almost at the bulge between the recti muscles, support the recti muscles with your hands, and pull them in and together.

5   Slowly lower your head.

3. WHEN KEGEL EXERCISES REALLY START TO MAKE SENSE

Reconnecting with your pelvic floor

• • •

It takes a little thing like pregnancy and childbirth to open your eyes to the fact that you actually have a pelvic floor, the thin layer of muscle that supports the vagina, rectum, bladder, and the other organs of the pelvis and abdomen. And that's only because everywhere you turn, somebody is reminding you to strengthen it.

While you were pregnant you probably thought a lot about doing pelvic floor exercises, encouraged, no doubt, by the promise of an easier labor and delivery; a swifter healing process; a future not overshadowed by adult diapers; and a lifetime of increased sexual sensation (in the unlikely event that you ever felt like having sex again).

And all the while, the softening hormones of your pregnancy, coupled with the new weight you were carrying, conspired to put an increased workload on these muscles as your once-taut (there's that word again) pelvic floor began to bow like an overly laden shelf. And all the while, pretty much unintentionally, you found better things to do with your pelvic floor than contract it. You took it to the movies; you made dinner together; the two of you picked out a color scheme for your baby's bedroom.

After all that, you can only imagine what kind of state your pelvic floor is in now, especially if you had a vaginal delivery, with all the stretching that it entails (not to mention the potential for an episiotomy).

Let's assume, just for the heck of it, that you've never really exercised your pelvic floor before now. (If you have, you have our permission to move on to the next chapter as long as you promise to contract while you're turning the pages.) Your first task is to learn how to isolate these muscles.

Here's how: Imagine you are in a public place and (heaven forbid) you suddenly start peeing (this is far more likely now that you have given birth to a baby, by the way). Clearly, you would use every resource at your disposal to stop the flow. Those resources have a name: pelvic floor muscles. Or *Kegels,* in honor of Dr. Arnold Kegel, a professor of obstetrics and gynecology at the University of California in Los Angeles, who exhibited an unusual but ultimately useful interest in the pelvic floor.

Now that you know where they are, here's what you should do with them. The following exercises are variations on a theme. To begin with, get comfortable with the first one, Your Basic Pelvic Floor Exercise. Practice this one frequently—every time you're waiting for a stoplight to change, for example, or while you're standing in line at the store. It's also wise, at this early postpartum stage, to contract your pelvic floor muscles any time you strain (like when you lift your baby) or when you sneeze or cough. Just a friendly warning.

EXERCISE: YOUR BASIC PELVIC FLOOR EXERCISE
Frequency: Ten times a day

Note: Your abdominals, buttocks, and inner thighs should be relaxed and your breathing normal. Start slowly and increase the repetitions gradually.

1   Lie down on your back or side, with your knees bent and your arms resting comfortably on the surface below you.

2   On the count of one, slowly tighten your pelvic floor muscles.

3   On the count of two, increase the tension in the muscles as you concentrate on *lifting up* and *drawing in.*

4   On the count of three, increase the tension in your muscles even higher.

5   On the count of four, strive for the highest degree of muscle tension you can. Hold this tension for a count of four.

6   Release this tension as you count slowly backward from four to one.
    Don't be dismayed if you can't do this slow release for the count of four—it's
    just a matter of practice.

When you've mastered the basics, try the Elevator and the Hammock.

EXERCISE: THE ELEVATOR
Frequency: Ten times a day

1   Lie on your back or side in bed or on an exercise mat. Imagine that your
    vaginal opening is an elevator door and the vaginal canal is an elevator shaft.

2   Using your pelvic floor muscles, slowly close the elevator doors for a
    count of four.

3   Then slowly tighten the muscles inside your vagina in an upward motion,
    as if you were lifting the elevator. Continue to slowly lift your imaginary
    elevator to the first floor, then to the second floor, and then to the third floor.

4   Slowly release the elevator in reverse order.

When this becomes too easy, try taking the elevator to the first floor,
open the elevator doors, close them, and then go up to the next floor. And so on.

EXERCISE: THE HAMMOCK
Frequency: Ten times a day

1   Visualize your pelvic floor muscles as a sling of muscles that form a hammock
    from your pubic bone in the front of your pelvis to your tailbone at the back.

2   Starting at the front tip of this hammock and working toward the back, slowly
    contract your pelvic floor muscles. The entire muscular sling should be tight
    by the time you've reached the tip of the hammock attached to your tailbone.

3   Slowly release the tension in your muscles from front to back.

4. IT ONLY HURTS WHEN I MOVE/ LAUGH/STAND UP STRAIGHT

The importance of posture

• • •

Over forty weeks your body gradually stretched and expanded to accommodate a slowly growing baby. But, suddenly, there's no baby to accommodate. And with no baby to act as ballast for your body, your whole internal abdominal and pelvic area has to work exceptionally hard to adapt to this abrupt change in circumstances and return to its pre-pregnancy status quo.

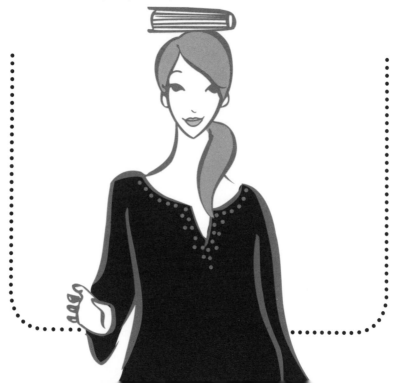

As your body has been used to counterbalancing the extra weight around your middle, a lack of baby may also cause you to hunch forward—a tendency that's exacerbated by your new tasks. Each new day finds you feeding, holding, changing, lifting, and carrying a baby that's getting increasingly rounder, fatter, and heavier. As anybody who's ever played Jenga knows, adding weight to a less-than-stable posture causes problems. With the newly postpartum human female, these problems usually take the form of neck, shoulder, and back pain.

Check your posture.

You can take action against these irritations and agonies by working on optimal postural alignment. Start by imagining that all the bones of your spine and your skull are threaded onto a string that, thanks to gravity and probably some other complex laws of physics, falls perfectly perpendicular to the ground, bringing your spine into equally perfect alignment.

While this may be a natural position for your spine, given your current muscle tension, years of bad habits, and recent pregnancy, it probably won't come naturally quite yet. But you can take a step in the right direction by practicing the following straightforward exercises.

Both the Seated Posture Check and the Standing Posture Check exercises on the following page will help you align your spine properly and engage the muscles that support it. Be diligent in doing these exercises every time you are either sitting or standing with your baby—you'll be getting a great workout and improving your posture almost without knowing it. It'll also help you focus more intently on bringing your abdominals and pelvic floor muscles back into line, while reducing stress on your shoulders and neck.

EXERCISE: SEATED POSTURE CHECK

Frequency: As often as possible

This simple (no sweating required) posture exercise can really help you feel tall, counteracting the negative effects of your new daily routines. Practice it consistently—every time you sit down with your baby—for the next three days, and you'll feel the results.

1   Hold your baby, and sit on a chair with your legs uncrossed.

2   Position your weight evenly over both buttocks.

3   Contract your pelvic floor muscles, draw your abdominal muscles in, and imagine stacking each vertebra from your pelvic floor on up, right through the crown of your head.

4   Drop your shoulders away from your ears, and lift your chin up and away from your chest. If you want to look down at your baby, do so by lowering your eyes, not by moving your neck.

EXERCISE: STANDING POSTURE CHECK

Frequency: As often as possible

Like the Seated Posture Check, this simple exercise will help lengthen and realign your spine. Try it first without your baby. Then, when you've mastered the technique and feel ready to kick things up a notch, introduce your baby into the routine.

1   Stand up straight on a firm, flat surface.

2   Imagine that each foot has four corners—inside and outside, toes and heel— and evenly distribute your weight across all four points on both feet.

3   With your feet as solid as possible, lengthen your legs, draw inward the muscles you use for your pelvic floor exercises, and imagine that your hip bones are headlights shining directly forward.

4   Draw your belly muscles in, and mentally begin to stack each of your vertebrae one on top of the other, until you reach the top of your head.

5   As you do so, allow your shoulders to pull open and away from your ears, keeping your head as the very highest part of your body.

And tilt your pelvis.
● ● ●

As you work on developing perfect posture, you can ease your aching back muscles—especially those of the lower spine—with a little pelvic tilt. Pelvic tilts are great exercises for any time your back feels sore and tired (i.e., most of the time), as they use your abdominal muscles to pull your pelvis up and your buttocks to pull your pelvis down, thus flattening the hollow in the lower part of your spine and realigning your vertebrae.

There are four different pelvic tilts described on the following pages. We recommend that you start with Pelvic Tilt #1, as lying on your back is the easiest way to begin. But feel free to try them all and see which one feels most comfortable to you.

EXERCISE: PELVIC TILT #1 (THE ONE YOU DO ON THE FLOOR)
Frequency: Ten times a day

1   Lie on your back with your knees bent and your arms comfortably behind your head or at your side. Your shoulders and lower spine should be touching the floor at all times.

2   Inhale.

3   As you exhale, roll the lower tip of your pelvis up and the part of your pelvis that's closest to your waist down. You'll know that you're doing this right if the amount of space between your back and the floor decreases.

4   Inhale.

5   Exhale, and roll your pelvis, contract your abdominal muscles, and tighten your buttocks. Hold this position for three seconds, and then relax.

EXERCISE: PELVIC TILT #2 (THE ONE YOU DO ON YOUR SIDE)
Frequency: Ten times a day

1   Lie on your side, a pillow or your hands under your head, your knees bent softly.

2   Inhale, releasing your abdominal muscles.

3   Exhale, and tip the lower portion of your pelvis forward and the top backward.

4   Inhale, and release your abdominal muscles.

5   Exhale, and on the outward breath tip your pelvis, contract your abdominals, and tighten your buttocks. Hold for three seconds, and then relax.

EXERCISE: PELVIC TILT #3 (THE ONE YOU DO STANDING UP)

Frequency: Ten times a day

1   Stand up with your toes pointing forward and your knees slightly bent. Your weight should be supported evenly on both feet.

2   Relax your shoulders, and keep them parallel to the floor.

3   Inhale.

4   As you exhale, curl your spine into a C shape with your pelvis tucked under; release.

EXERCISE: PELVIC TILT #4 (THE ONE YOU DO WITH A CHAIR)

Frequency: Ten times a day

1   Stand with your feet comfortably apart and your toes pointing in opposite directions as you hold onto the back of a chair.

2   Inhale, and lower yourself four or five inches by bending at the knees.

3   Exhale as you come back up, tucking your buttocks under and pulling up on your abdominal muscles. Hold this position for ten seconds. Release.

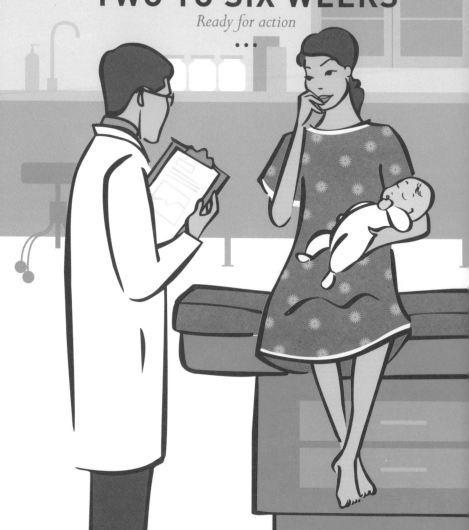

CHAPTER 3

TWO TO SIX WEEKS

Ready for action

. . .

Your baby's just a couple of weeks old, and already you're on the third chapter. You're making amazing progress, and this is where things start to settle down. (At least on the exercise front—we can't take any responsibility for that child of yours and her erratic sleep schedule.)

At this point we're assuming that you're *au fait* with the basics—that you've mastered those all-important abdominals, pelvic floor, and posture-specific exercises. There's a reason why we devoted pages and pages to these exercises: it's so that by the time you get here, your body's in good shape to move forward. There is most definitely an order and a method to the way you need to approach a postpartum exercise program. Which is a roundabout way of saying that if you haven't read the earlier part of this book, go back and read it now.

If the last two chapters were all about preparing your body for exercise, this chapter is all about getting the green light to go for it. Here, you'll learn more about what happens at your first postpartum doctor's appointment (and there are some handy hints about the kind of questions you should be asking). We'll introduce you to some of the important philosophies that underpin any fitness program. There's an all-important stretching lesson (the first half of which you can actually do lying down) and then some thoughts on choosing the best kind of exercise class for you and your oh-so-demanding offspring.

This is an exciting place to be—you're on the cusp of putting all that good theory into energetic practice. And that means that you're almost a fit mama.

• • •

1. SO I'M BACK TO NORMAL, RIGHT?

Your first postpartum OB-GYN visit

• • •

So, you thought that after delivering that baby you were done with visiting your favorite medical establishment. Au contraire. Depending on your practitioner's preference and the type of birth experience you had, he or she will ask you to return for a checkup somewhere between two and six weeks later. This is a good thing, but just in case you're slightly nervous, here's what you can expect.

If you had a vaginal delivery, your practitioner will check your uterus (to make sure that it has returned, or is returning, to its normal size), your perineum (especially if you had stitches because of tearing or an episiotomy), and your breasts (whether or not you are breast-feeding). You may also have a blood test if you lost a large amount of blood during delivery. If you had a cesarean birth, your doctor will also make sure your incision is healing nicely.

But regardless of the type of delivery, you'll also be asked how you are feeling—if you have any concerns about your physical state of health or your emotional well-being. If you are feeling overwhelmed by your new role, or even just a little low, a little weepy, a little discombobulated, you should most definitely speak up.

And if you have any concerns or questions about the actual birth, ask away. You may not have cause to visit your doctor or midwife for months to come, so this may be your last opportunity to say what's on your mind before said mind becomes cluttered with the traumas and delights of child rearing. If, for example, you were disappointed that you had an epidural or you're not sure why you had an episiotomy, it's important that you voice your concerns—not least because you may very well find yourself giving birth to another baby at some point in the not-so-distant future.

Aside from confirming your physical and emotional health, your doctor will probably raise a few questions.

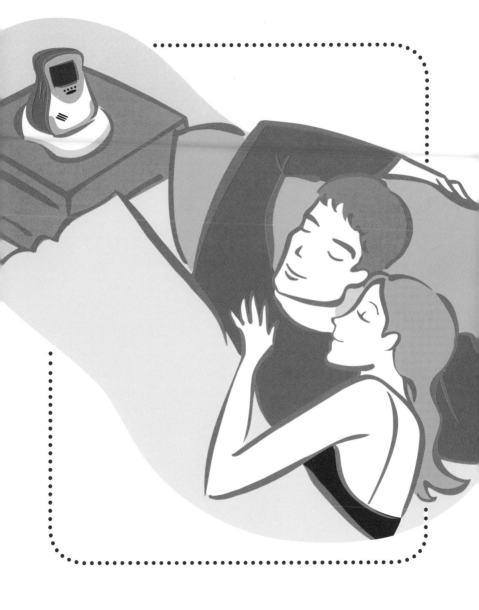

The question of sex.
• • •

You'll find that most practitioners will recommend six weeks of what is gently referred to as *pelvic rest*. This period of (probably not unwelcome) celibacy is designed to give your pelvic area time to heal and your cervix a chance to close. Then, whether you are even remotely interested in the notion or not, your doctor will bring up the question of sex. (Apparently he or she is looking for some repeat business from you.)

It's natural to have some concerns about your future sex life. Does it, for example, even have a future? You may be worried that sex will be uncomfortable or painful; that you'll be too tired to enjoy it or initiate it; that you're not really interested anyway; that now you're breast-feeding, your breasts are off-limits (and that's going to be pretty unpopular); that you're still bleeding; and/or that your baby will wake up at a critical juncture. All these fears are more than normal, and all will fade over time as your hormones stabilize and as you get used to being a mom (and get really, really good at [a] multitasking, and [b] keeping everybody happy).

If it makes you feel any better, know that your partner has at least as many concerns. Your partner may be worried that sex will cause you pain; that you'll leak milk from your breasts (which you probably will and which you may even find amusing); that you don't enjoy the things you used to enjoy; and/or that you're no longer interested in sex. (Some men may feel especially uncomfortable, even turned off, after seeing their partner give birth. While unusual, this is also fairly serious and requires professional help.)

If you or your partner do have any concerns, start by talking to each other. It's also a good idea to bite the bullet and have sex sooner rather than later (by which point the specter of what feels like losing your virginity again will have become a behemoth). If sex is uncomfortable (and it probably will be at first), then practice other ways of enjoying intimacy. Take things slowly, and be sure to use a water-soluble lubricant, as vaginal dryness is a normal part of postpartum life.

One of the biggest fears surrounding sex—a fear that will probably strike both of you with equal horror—is that you might get pregnant again. Your practitioner will probably anticipate this fear, as evidenced by his/her second big question.

The question of birth control.
• • •
You may not believe it now, but people do go on to have sex after having a baby and, consequently, quite often go on to have another baby. If one is enough for you at the moment, thank you very much, listen carefully to your doctor or midwife. It's true, breast-feeding can suppress the return of ovulation for months, but it's not a fool-proof contraceptive. There's no harm in having a backup plan, and there are many birth control options that are safe to practice while breast-feeding. Your doctor will be happy to advise you. Even if you're on the fence about intimacy right now, assume that (not to mix metaphors or anything) you'll be back in the saddle at some point, and take the opportunity to discuss your options with your practitioner.

While your doctor will talk about sex and about contraception, he or she will most likely overlook the other big question.

The question of exercise.
• • •
Many doctors tell their new-mom patients that they shouldn't exercise for six weeks after the birth. No offense to your doctor, who we're sure is quite lovely, but this is wrong. It doesn't mean that your doctor is incompetent, just slightly ill-informed. Most obstetricians are so focused on nurturing the pregnant woman and safely delivering her baby that their postpartum care of the same woman tends to take a backseat. The bottom line is this: if you had a normal and safe delivery and your postpartum checkup confirms that you are healing well, then there is absolutely no reason why you shouldn't embark on a postpartum exercise program. Sorry, ladies—not even medical opinion can get you out of this one.

2. I WILL ALWAYS DRINK WATER BEFORE I EXERCISE

And other important fitness mantras

• • •

If there's a little corner of your brain that isn't filled with thoughts of diaper absorbency, car seat installation instructions, and strategies for finagling a babysitter, use it to store away the following important fitness philosophies.

I will have mastered my restorative exercises well before I get to page 95.
• • • •

You're ready to go. Your doctor has given you the all clear for takeoff, and you're currently on course for a more vigorous exercise program that will include cardio, strength training, and flexibility components. And you're quite the expert when it comes to your restorative pelvic floor, abdominal, and posture exercises. Don't flake on these components; while it's tempting to flip to the back of the book, if you don't master the basics, you're not going to be in any kind of shape to start kickboxing.

I will dress comfortably for exercise.
• • • •

Starting an exercise program is also a great excuse to go shopping and treat yourself to something fun and sporty (not to mention stretchy). And as we recommend that you dress in layers so you can peel off according to the temperature (yours), you'll probably want to buy lots.

I will always wear a supportive bra.
• • • •

If you're breast-feeding, you'll need to wear an extremely supportive bra (or two) when you exercise. If your breasts tend to leak milk, use breast pads and change them often so as to keep excess moisture away from the nipple tissue, as this can cause cracks and infection.

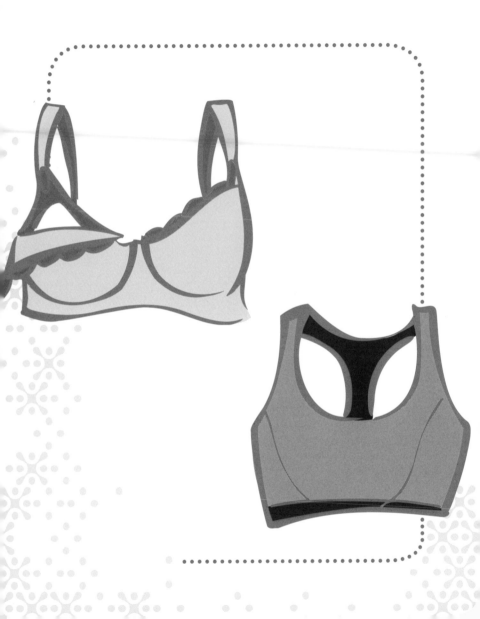

I will wear suitable footwear.

● ● ● ●

This means supportive shoes for cardio, running, or gym exercising, or bare feet if yoga or Pilates is your exercise of choice.

I will always accessorize appropriately.

● ● ● ●

If you're exercising outside, slather on the sunscreen and bring an extra tube with you. Figure out some way to carry everything on your person (like a fanny pack) or stuff it all in your overstuffed diaper bag or stroller if your baby is accompanying you. Also, think about investing in some manner of personal entertainment system. (Music can be very motivating, and at this stage in the game you may need some extra motivation.)

I will learn to find exercise equipment quite fascinating.

● ● ● ●

If you're doing yoga, invest in a good yoga mat. (They're different from regular exercise mats and less slippery.) Other accessories that you might consider buying include a physical therapy ball, weights (two-, three-, or five-pound ones), and resistance bands. All can be used comfortably in your own home, and a physical therapy ball makes a great adult-sized bouncy chair for when you're holding a cranky baby.

I will be flexible about my exercise schedule.

● ● ● ●

You may intend to exercise on a regular basis, but it's not always so easy to put theory into practice. Remember that baby and her ever-so-unpredictable sched-ule? Just as it affects when you sit down to a meal (at unsociable hours) or get to bed (way past bedtime), it's going to affect when you are able to get to a class (two hours later). Thus, it's a good idea to have an open, flexible attitude to your exercise schedule. Or, even better, have a Plan B or two up your sleeves. This could be an exercise DVD for your personal, in-home gym (i.e., your living room); a brisk walk up and down a few hills; or the ability to accept, without feeling guilty, that this morning is just not going to be the right time to work out. Always keep your options open: while you may prefer your indoor exercise class, there are organized classes that meet outdoors that may be more appealing to your baby. Be flexible, be prepared to shift gears, and always assure your offspring that she's not getting out of the workout *that* easily.

And I will always drink water before I exercise.
• • • •
Adequate hydration is important for anybody exercising. It's particularly important for you, as thermoregulation can be an issue for new moms. It will also help avoid (or lessen) constipation, reduce hemorrhoids, and keep your skin glowing. Start chugging.

3. HOW HIGH CAN YOU GO (WITHOUT CAFFEINE)?

Stop hunching, start stretching

• • •

Stretching. It seems so simple, doesn't it? After all, you've been doing it for years and years now, and with every sign of success. Why, only this morning you dragged your reluctant body out of bed and indulged in a nice big stretch right there and then.

But the truth is, there's more to stretching than meets the eye. And wouldn't you know it, there's a right way and wrong way to stretch. It's important to get stretching right, as it helps to improve your flexibility, one of the major measures of physical fitness, and protect your joints. So now that you've gotten super-good at what we call *base camp exercises* (the abdominal, pelvic, and postural exercises we discussed in chapter 2), it's time to stretch some. Here's more on why you should spend some real time and effort here.

Why you should stretch.
• • •
We all know that stretching warms up the body to prepare it for more vigorous exercise. But that's not all. Stretching also increases coordination and kinesthetic awareness; decreases muscle tension; increases blood flow to the working muscles; lubricates the joints that move the muscles; elongates and aligns the spine; and is simply a good-feeling way to get the kinks out. Whew. Remember, a truly healthy muscle is one that not only contracts well (demonstrating strength and endurance) but also relaxes well (showing flexibility). Stretching helps you do both.

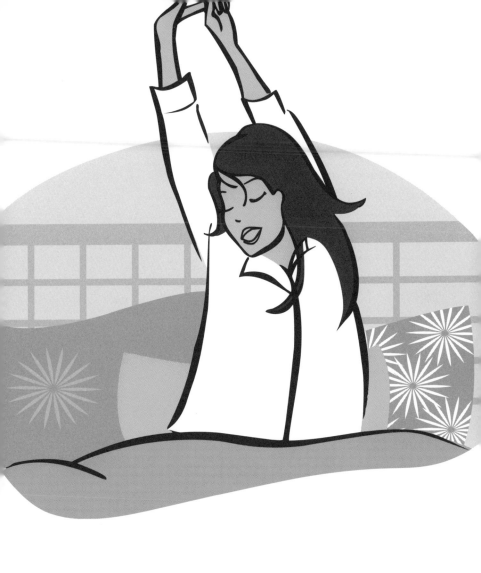

When you should stretch.
• • • •

The short answer is *anytime*. The slightly longer answer is before exercise, after exercise, after hunching over to feed your baby, after contorting your body to carry unnecessarily heavy baby equipment (and/or baby), and before you go to bed (or collapse on the sofa).

What you should stretch.
• • • •

The short answer is *everything*. And the slightly longer answer is all your major muscle groups, especially those that are under- or overused.

How you should stretch.
• • •

Slow and *steady* should be your watchwords. Never bounce; always hold your stretch; and always release it slowly.

That was Stretching 101. Think you passed? Now it's time to put theory into practice. The good news is that there's no better position in which to stretch than lying down. It's a great way to do all that important lengthening and strengthening of the spine that will create basic support of all of the following stretches.

The following Full-Body Stretch warms up every major muscle group. We've broken it up into *eight* manageable sections (yes, there really is that much stretching that you should be doing) to make it easier to understand, but the stretch should be attempted as o*ne continuous sequence*. So no sneaking off to make yourself a cup of tea between Part 5 and Part 6.

EXERCISE: THE FULL-BODY STRETCH

Frequency: Once before exercising or whenever you don't have time for a full workout session

Part 1

1   Lie down on a firm, flat surface with your knees bent and the soles of your feet together.

2   Allow your knees to gently fall away from each other.

3   Hold this position for thirty seconds or longer.

4   Extend your arms out to the sides with your palms facing up.

5   Slowly and gently roll your head from side to side. Repeat five times.

6   With your head facing to the right, gently nod your head up and down. Repeat five times.

7   Repeat step 6 with your head facing to the left.

Part 2

1   Bring your knees together so that your inner thighs are touching.

2   Loosely clasp your hands below your knees, and allow your lower back to drop gently toward the floor. Remember to keep your abdominal muscles engaged.

3   Inhale, relax your neck, and exhale while gently pulling your knees in toward your chest.

4   Hold this position while focusing on your breathing.

5   Bring your chin toward your chest.

6   Lower your head to the floor.

Part 3

1. With your knees still pulled up to your chest, slowly roll them in a circle five times clockwise. Repeat counterclockwise.

2. Release your left leg, and lower it to the floor.

3. Gently stretch your right leg up to the ceiling, and hold this position for five slow, deep breaths.

4. Then, circle your right foot from the ankle five times clockwise and five times counterclockwise. Release your knee, bend your leg, and lower it to its starting position against your chest.

5. Gently grasp the outside of this knee with your left hand, and slowly pull your entire right leg all the way across your abdomen to the left side of your body.

6. Extend your right arm out to your right side, and gently turn your head toward it. Hold this position for as long as you want, as you focus on your breathing.

7. Bring your right knee back to your chest, extend it, and lower it to the floor. Rest.

8. Repeat this sequence with your left leg.

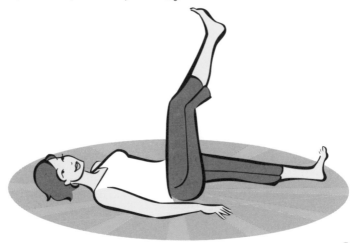

Part 4

1 Position yourself on your hands and knees. Your knees should be directly below your hips, with your elbows and wrists lined up below your shoulders.

2 Inhale, and release your lower back into a gentle swayback position.

3 Exhale, and bring your chin to your chest. Round your back like an angry cat.

4 Repeat five times.

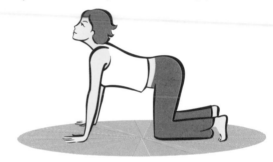

Part 5

1 Slowly come up into a standing position.

2 Be sure your feet are firmly planted on the floor. (As you did with the Standing Posture Check on page 68, think of your feet as having four corners—inside of the tip of the big toe; outside of the tip of the little toe; outside corner of the heel; inside corner of the heel. Try to distribute your body's weight evenly over each corner.)

3 Imagine you're trying to push the weight of your body through the center of the earth.

4 From here, imagine lengthening your body from your feet through the inside of your calves, knees, inner thighs, and pelvic floor, and through the outside of your calves, thighs, and buttocks.

5 Draw your pelvic floor muscles in with a Kegel contraction, and pull in your abdominal muscles toward your spine.

6 Relax your shoulders away from your ears, and open your rib cage. You should feel a slight opening through your upper back.

7   Relax your neck, and visualize the top of your head as an extension of a long line that runs from the middle of the space between your feet, through your pelvis, abdominal muscles, and right up to the sky. Stay in this stance as you take several deep abdominal breaths. (See page 61 if you need an Abdominal Breathing refresher.)

Part 6

1   Inhale, and gently reach your arms out away from your body and up over your head, pushing your shoulders away from your ears.

2   Bring the palms of your hands together, so that your index fingers reach up to the sky, with your other fingers clasped around each other.

3   Tighten and extend your arms over your head, still keeping your shoulders away from your ears.

4   Inhale, exhale, and gently lean to your left. Concentrate on pulling your abdominal muscles *in* and your pelvic floor muscles *up*; hold this position for fifteen seconds. Remember to keep breathing as you hold this stretch.

5   Inhale, and exhale as you return your body to a centered, upright position.

6   Inhale, and repeat on the right side of your body.

7   Repeat this part five times.

Part 7

1   Drop your arms to your sides, and slowly roll your shoulders back five times and forward five times.

2   Repeat this sequence five times.

3   Slowly shrug your shoulders up and down five times. Be sure to focus on the downward part of the stretch.

Part 8

1   Inhale, and bring your arms up over your head.

2   Exhale, and "swan dive" your arms down to the floor in a forward fold (or as close to it as you can comfortably go). Your knees can be slightly bent if this is easier for you.

3   Focus on your breathing and lengthening your spine. Let your head and neck relax.

4   Hold as you inhale and exhale at least five times.

5   Inhale, soften your knees, and using the strength of your abdominal muscles, slowly uncurl vertebra by vertebra until you are back in the starting standing position.

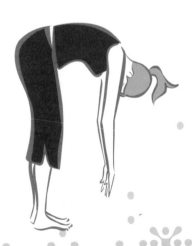

4. KICKBOXING OR TAI CHI?

Finding the perfect class for both of you

• • •

It's like the first day of a sale. Or looking at the dessert menu. Or picking out a stroller. Sometimes there are just too many choices. So while your body might be completely ready to start a more rigorous exercise program, when it comes to actually choosing an exercise class, your mind comes to a standstill, utterly confounded by the number of possibilities. Do you want to dial it down with tai chi, yoga, or Pilates? Or pump it up with cross-training, cycling, or kickboxing? Do you want to head to the hills for a run? Or hit the gym for an aerobics or step class? It's enough to make even the most determined wannabe fitness maven curl up on the couch in the fetal position.

Work through your dilemma, slowly and surely, by asking yourself the following pertinent questions.

Q: What kind of class should I try?

A: Do something that you like doing. You're much more likely to keep at it if you choose an activity you enjoy. Or opt for something you've always wanted to try. After all, this is the time for new experiences.

Q: What should I look for in a class?

A: Any class you choose should include a proper warm-up and elements of cardio-vascular activity, strength training, and stretching. Your class should be taught to various fitness levels. It should be mindful of, and be able to adapt to, where you are in the postpartum return to fitness continuum.

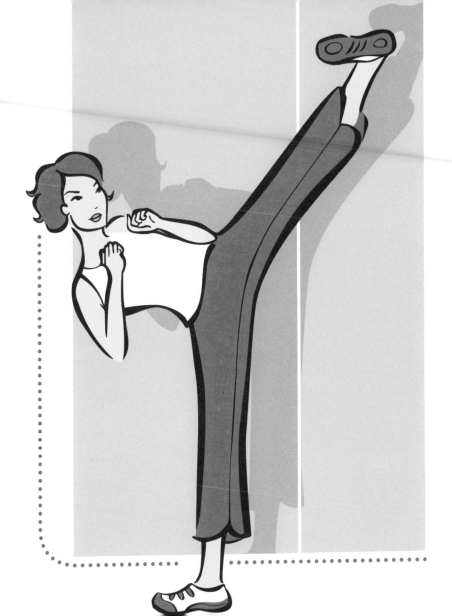

Q: How will I find the perfect class?

A: Shop around, and try out a class or two. Take advantage of those complimentary first class offers, and you'll be exercising for free. And don't forget to ask other moms. There are all manner of places where you'll meet your own kind—your doctor's office, your pediatrician's office, the park, baby stores. Use the people you meet as sources of information (about anything, really, not just exercise classes).

Q: How will I maintain the momentum?

A: Find a workout buddy—it's more fun, and you'll increase your chances of making it to class if someone is expecting you (and will harass you without mercy if you don't arrive).

Q: What about my baby?

A: Find a class that is baby-friendly or, even better, baby-centered, like a stroller-based class (because a baby is clearly a requirement), or create your own with a group of moms you can stroll with on a regular basis. Alternatively, look for a fitness center that offers day care facilities. Many centers won't take babies under three months, so remember to read the fine print. If all else fails, find a class you can do at a time of day your partner or a friend can watch your baby.

One of the best ways to meet all of the above requirements is to find a specially designated postpartum exercise class. Here's why.

You can take your baby.

Not to state the obvious, but your baby will generally be welcome. This will make life easier for you and is a great way for your baby to start socializing with children his own age.

It's geared to your unique physical needs.

The instructor will have had special training (be sure to check his or her credentials) and will know the best way to whip those postpartum muscles into action.

It's an easy way to advance your fitness routine.

Once you've completed this class, you can graduate to the next level of postpartum class offered.

It's a great way to meet other mothers.

And why shouldn't your exercise routine be fun?

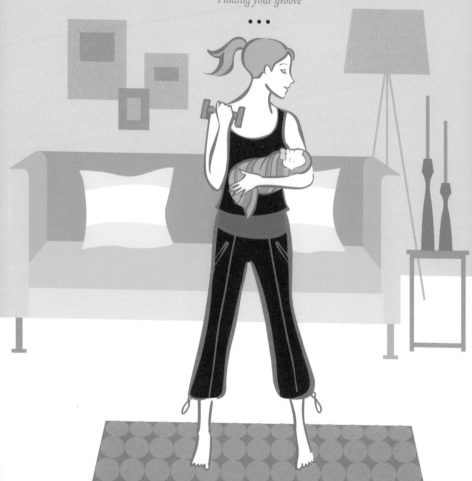

CHAPTER 4

SIX WEEKS
TO SIX MONTHS

Finding your groove

. . .

There's a big difference between six weeks and six months postpartum, but at some point between the two you'll start to realize that you're enjoying getting fit and that you're actually finding it a little easier than you did a few weeks ago. Whether this happens closer to six weeks or to six months really doesn't matter; simply know that it will happen, and glory in any progress you make along the way.

When it does happen, it's time to think about introducing strength training and aerobic components into your workout. In this chapter, you'll learn more about each activity and how you can include either (and preferably both) into your exercise regimen. But let's start with a quick word of warning—it's very important that your pelvic floor and abdominal muscles are in good shape before introducing any degree of aerobic activity into your workout, so if those areas aren't sufficiently strengthened, please stop right here and go back to chapter 2.

If you're getting bored with your solitary approach to exercise, you'll also see how you can spin it a couple of other ways, either by integrating your baby into your fitness routine (well, if you've got a weight on hand, you might as well use it) or by exercising with a group. There are real advantages to both, and we advise you to make every effort to explore them as you find your own personal exercise groove.

• • •

1. IF YOU CAN DELIVER A BABY, THIS SHOULD BE A SNAP

Why you already have the strength for strength training

• • •

You've already proved that you're a superstrong being. You carried that big baby-filled belly around for the best part of a year and labored long and hard to introduce your child to the world. And you spent the last few weeks with a steadily growing lump of a baby attached to your arm/shoulder/boob. You are one powerful woman.

All this is very good preparation for introducing strength training—a more systematic approach to building muscle and improving overall physical strength—into your fitness regimen. But if you balk at the thought of bulking up, remember that huge muscles (and a propensity to wear a teeny-weeny bikini barely covering your supremely tanned and oiled body) are not a necessary consequence of this type of activity. If you need further convincing, note that there are some excellent reasons why everybody, especially postpartum women, should incorporate strength training into a fitness routine.

- **Do it for your bones.** It's a fact that strength training can increase bone density and help prevent osteoporosis later in life.

- **Do it for your muscles.** If your muscles are showing a distinct lack of tautness, it may not be your baby's fault (well, not exclusively). Everybody's muscle mass is on a downward trajectory once we get past our early twenties, and strength training is a great way to build 'em up and keep 'em strong.

- **Do it to increase your metabolism.** Strength training creates more lean muscle tissue, which helps speed up your metabolism. This, in turn, increases the number of calories you burn. And we all know what that means.

- **Do it for your back.** If you suffer from lower back pain (and why wouldn't you, what with all that lifting and carrying and bending over?), strength training may help ease your discomfort by increasing lower back strength and relieving stress on your posture.

Knowing you're already accomplished at the most important strength training exercises—those focused on your pelvic floor and abdomen—should spur you on to bigger and better things. Get yourself some free weights or resistance bands, plan on fifteen minutes a day, maybe three or four times a week, and be sure to follow these guidelines.

- **Stretch before and after.** Now that you're down with the Full-Body Stretch (see page 85 if you need a quick reminder), remember to add it on to either end of every single exercise session.

- **Start slowly.** Whatever kind of strength training exercise you do, start with twelve to fifteen repetitions. And just one set is fine for now, before working up to two or three sets.

- **Keep it light.** Make sure that any weight you work with is not so heavy that you can't do about a dozen repetitions without feeling like your arm is going to drop off. If you find yourself struggling, choose a lighter weight. (Of course, this is not to say that you should choose one that you could lift with your little finger.)

- **Concentrate on your breathing.** Be sure to exhale as you exert any force—that means on the hard part of any repetition.

- **Stop if it hurts.** This is a pretty good rule for almost anything to do with exercise. If you find yourself in pain or if you are experiencing symptoms such as faintness, dizziness, nausea, or extreme fatigue, stop. Take a break. Drink some water. Lie down.

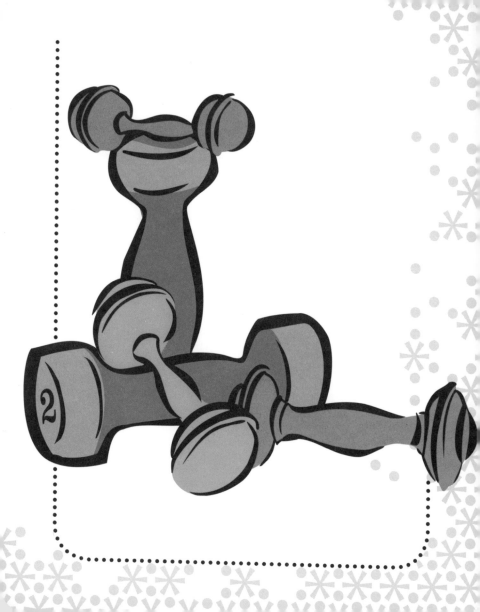

Here's a couple of simple weight training exercises, just to get you started.

EXERCISE: BICEP CURL
Frequency: Ten times with each arm

You'll need a couple of two-pound hand weights for this one.

1   Hold a weight in each hand, and stand with your feet hip-width apart.

2   Let your arms hang down at your sides with your palms facing in.

3   Draw in your abdominal muscles, and raise your right arm, bending at the elbow so your hand touches your shoulder. (You'll need to rotate your hand 90 degrees.)

4   Lower your arm slowly.

5   Repeat with your left arm.

EXERCISE: SHOULDER LIFT
Frequency: Ten times with each arm

This exercise requires a resistance band (sold in sports stores).

1   Stand with your feet together.

2   Take one pace forward with your left foot; place this foot on one end of the resistance band.

3   Hold the other end of the resistance band in your right hand.

4   Lean over until your torso is at an angle of about 45 degrees, contracting your abdominals as you do so.

5   Keep your right elbow slightly bent, and slowly raise your arm up to shoulder height.

6   Return your arm to its starting position, and repeat.

2. WORK IT, BABY

Energy-boosting, butt-firming aerobics

• • •

The fact that you're reading this section right now tells us—assuming that you're working through this book in a nice, orderly fashion—that you've absorbed the information about working on your abdominals and pelvic floor and that those particular muscle groups of yours are in fine fettle.

As we start to talk about aerobic exercise, there's nothing more important. Aerobic exercise can be great, but, particularly as a new mom, you have to be in a certain kind of shape to do it—and to do it without suffering the consequences. For, yes, there are certain intrinsic dangers associated with the donning of workout gear if you haven't already paid due attention to your postpartum pelvic floor and abdominal muscles.

We have just two words for you—*urinary* and *incontinence*.

That's because traditional aerobic exercise (especially in the Jane Fonda sense of the term) incorporates erratic and bouncing movements, which can place undue stress on weakened and poorly conditioned pelvic floor muscles.

The good news is that you can still get the benefit of aerobic activity without *going for the burn*. After all, aerobic exercise is defined as any activity that makes your heart work faster and increases your breathing rate—not any activity that makes your heart work faster and requires that you spend a lot of money on exercise videos and leg warmers. And true *recreational aerobic exercise* (the kind that's gentler on your body) can be assimilated pretty easily into your daily life. Brisk walking is aerobic activity. (Slow walking is too, depending on your fitness level, lung capacity, and personal stamina.) Hiking and cycling are aerobic exercises. Swimming is great aerobic exercise.

But what's so good about it? Let's take a moment for a quick biology lesson.

Regular aerobic exercise helps improve your cardiovascular fitness—the ability of your lungs, heart, and vascular system to get oxygen to your muscles. The better they are at this, the more efficiently your body uses its oxygen supply. And when this happens, your heart doesn't have to work so hard to pump blood and oxygen around your body. And a stronger, more efficient heart is a good thing. The bottom line—aerobic exercise improves your circulatory and respiratory systems, increases your endurance, strengthens your muscles, and, as a not unuseful bonus, can help you lose weight.

Despite its obvious advantages, there are some things (i.e., some body parts) that you should consider carefully before you embark on an aerobic exercise program.

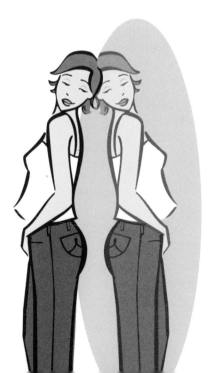

- **Your pelvic floor.** As we've said before, it's important that your pelvic floor is in good condition—especially if you insist on doing more traditional aerobics. That way, your body can take the extra bouncing around that's inevitable if you run or take a moderately active class.

- **Your boobs.** They're bigger than before, especially if you're breast-feeding. While this fact is probably hard to ignore on a daily basis, large boobs are even more, er, *in your face* when you're trying to do aerobic exercise.

- **Your joints.** Levels of *relaxin*—the joint-softening hormone of pregnancy—return to normal just days after delivery, but your joints may be lax for up to three months later. Be careful to avoid sudden jumping motions that jar your body, as it's possible to overstretch and even dislocate these joints, especially your hip, back, and knees.

Perhaps more than any other form of exercise (not counting things like bungee jumping and parasailing), aerobic exercise has the potential to do harm to the new mom's new postpartum body. Take good care of yourself by sticking to the following guidelines.

- **Warm up every time.** Remember to warm up with some good stretches, like the Full-Body Stretch on page 85.

- **Get kitted out.** Invest in a really good pair of sneakers (get professionally fitted) and a decent bra (likewise).

- **Stay hydrated.** As with all forms of exercise, drink plenty of water before, during, and after.

- **Take it slowly.** This is not the time to be competitive—even with yourself. Give your body ample time in which to adjust to unfamiliar movements.

- **Think before you jump.** Avoid aerobic activity on hard surfaces, as they can be too jarring to your body. (Carpet, sprung floors, and grassy areas are better.)

- **Focus on non-weight-bearing aerobic exercise.** Try swimming and cycling. (Stationary cycling can be especially good.) Both activities help you build up your cardiovascular strength without putting undue stress on your joints.

- **Keep at it.** Cardiovascular exercise is most effective when done regularly, say, two or three times a week. That way, you'll build up joint strength over time, rather than shocking your poor body with the occasional but intense session.

- **Listen to your body.** As always, stop if you experience pain or feel faint, nauseous, or overly fatigued.

In the next chapter, we talk about more specific aerobic exercises. For now, though, your mission (if you choose to accept it) is to do some form of aerobic exercise every day. And a great way to do this is by walking. For at least fifteen minutes of your stroller-pushing day, pick up the pace, stand really tall, and walk with purpose toward that coffee shop.

3. MEET YOUR
NEW WORKOUT PARTNER

Exercising with your baby

• • •

One of the great things about exercising with a baby is that you get a naturally progressive workout. As you get fitter, your child gets a little heavier, and your workouts get more strenuous. It's a perfect system, really.

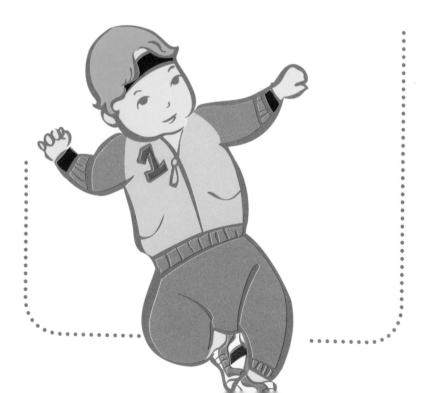

And it's a wonderful way to enjoy *productive* time with your child. If you're starting to feel like a walking boob whose only function is to attend to your child's every whim, making your baby a necessary part of your workout can help redress the balance somewhat, and this can only be good for your relationship.

Working out with your baby also counters one of the biggest obstacles to fitness for the new mom—the logistical matter of when and where. A baby, considering his small size, takes up a disproportionate amount of time and energy, and may severely compromise your ability to exercise when and how you want to. Incorporating your baby into your fitness plan is a great way to eliminate at least one of the stumbling blocks, although it does kind of override your formerly cast-iron excuse for not joining a friend for her evening constitutional ("Oh, I can't make it—I can't get a babysitter"). The key to exercising successfully with your baby is finding the right time to do it and the right place.

Pick your time.
• • •
Well, there's nap time, and there are other times. If your baby's nap time is the only time *you* get to grab forty winks, then develop some exercise routine in which your baby can be a willing—and alert—participant. An old disco mix on tape and a bouncy chair can be a great distraction for your small friend, and they allow you to develop a fitness session at home, with or without equipment.

Pick your place.
• • •
By the simple yet judicious introduction of different tactics and equipment, it's entirely possible to develop both an indoor and an outdoor baby-centric exercise routine. Here's how.

Outdoors. Exercising outside is fantastic for both of you. While it's easy to stay home—you don't have to pack the diaper bag, worry about overdressing your baby, or imagine the poopfest that will inevitably happen when it's least convenient—try to convince yourself that the advantages (fresh air, stimulation from a change of scenery, the personal satisfaction derived from actually getting out of the house) outweigh the slight inconveniences. And, if you have the budget, certain pieces of equipment can facilitate your new outdoor mom-and-baby exercise routines.

JOGGING STROLLER. Note: you don't have to jog while using it. A brisk walk can be just as effective and is much easier on your joints. Either way, it'll keep your baby well occupied (or lull him to sleep). Find a jogging stroller that reclines if your baby is less than six months or so; otherwise your regular stroller will do for walking (not running).

FRONT PACK. As well as keeping your baby nice and snug against you, a front pack is a good way of adding a little extra weight into your routine. It also necessitates a low-tech approach to exercise—no stroller, no bulky diaper bag, no unnecessary equipment. Just load her up, and off you go.

BACKPACK. Again, this is a great way to lift weights without realizing you're doing it. You can transition from the front pack to the backpack right around the six-month mark (or whenever your child can sit up unsupported).

Indoors. If you can't talk yourself into braving the outdoors, take a look at the following in-home mom-and-baby exercises. They're a great way to keep your baby occupied while you actually accomplish something. (This is ordinarily an impossibility, unless your baby is the kind of child who is really into vacuuming.)

EXERCISE: THE AMAZING, INCREDIBLE FLYING BABY!

Frequency: Twice a day

This is great for strengthening the arms, back, and chest and can soothe a fussing baby. When your baby is young, hold her so that she faces in toward your body; as she gets older, you can hold her facing away from you so that she enjoys a more interesting view (no offense).

1   Stand with your legs hip-width apart.

2   Hold your baby against your chest.

3   Inhale, exhale, and raise your baby to the right as you lean your body to the right.

4   Let your shoulders relax, keeping your chest open.

5   Repeat on the left side of your body.

6   Do one set of five—or more if your baby is enjoying the experience.

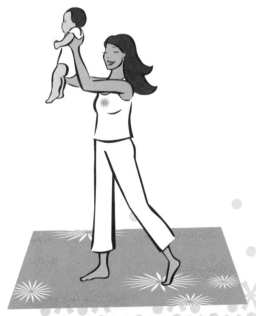

EXERCISE: BABY ON BOARD

Frequency: Twice a day

This one is great for strengthening the abdomen while toning the buttocks.

1   Lie on your back with your legs bent and off the ground.

2   Place your baby, belly down, on top of your shins, supporting him there
    with your hands.

3   Bring your head and neck off the floor. (If this causes any discomfort to your
    neck, you can simply leave your head on the floor.)

4   Feel your abdominal muscles engage.

5   Slowly push your legs away from your body, and then draw them back
    into your body.

6   Repeat ten times.

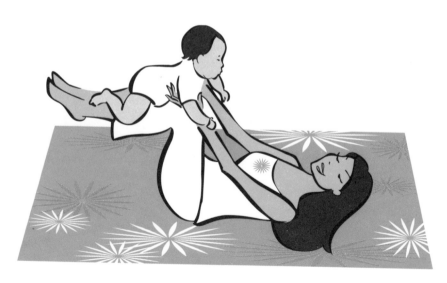

4. THE SISTERHOOD OF MOTHERHOOD

Why exercising with other moms is a great move

• • •

Not that you can't exercise solo—and some activities, like Kegel exercises, are most definitely a solitary event—but exercising with other new moms has some enormous advantages. And not all of them are directly concerned with fitness. Here are a few of our favorites.

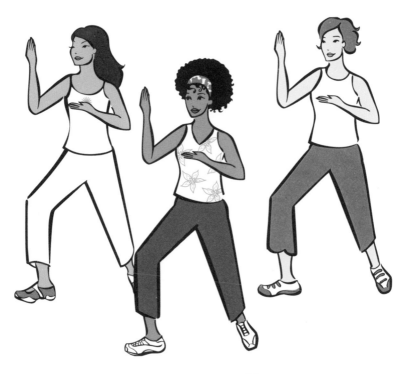

- **Healthy competition.** As a group, you and your fellow exercising moms will become pretty competitive about whose child is the smartest, whose butt is losing weight the fastest, whose stroller is the coolest—and who makes it to the top of the hill without having an asthma attack.

- **Motivation on tap.** When it's just you by your lonesome, it's easy to come up with excuses not to exercise *(Look at that pile of laundry!, My shoulder is feeling a little strained from when I bent down last night to get the ice cream out of the freezer,* or the perennial favorite, *I'm pacing myself).* Fortunately, your exercise posse won't swallow this kind of nonsense. They're there to encourage you, to cheer you on, and to otherwise get you fired up for victory over lethargy.

- **Automatic guilt-tripping.** And on the other end of the motivational spectrum—something you'll probably discover when you and your fellow moms know each other a little better—is the guilt-tripping that you get when you flake on a prearranged exercise session. But please don't resent their tough-love attitude. Your friends just have your best interests at heart. Either that or sleep deprivation is making them sadistic.

- **New friends.** You'll never be able to give up your old friends, but if those guys are more focused on office politics or the latest bar to try on a Friday night, you'll enjoy hanging out with women with whom you have something in common. Like babies. And compromised abdominals.

- **Babysitting connections.** As long as you're prepared to return the favor, the easiest people to hit up for babysitting are other people with babies. With an exercise group—even if it's only two or three of you—comes a ready supply of sitters who are every bit as eager as you are for a night off.

- **Ego boosting.** While you're immensely proud of your new baby, your new body perhaps just isn't quite there yet. All the other new moms know that you need a little flattery to make you feel good, and just as you compliment the gal next to you in the strollercise class on her fine leg extension, so you can expect return compliments on your ramrodlike posture.

- **Empathy on tap.** Who else understands the traumas of sleepless nights, impossibly large hemorrhoids, and not-helpful-enough partners like another new mom? Maybe your workout partners don't have all the answers to the meaning of your new life, but a trouble shared really is a trouble halved. Exercise in a group, and you can cut your issues down to size.

- **Confirmation that yours really is the most beautiful child. Ever.** Exercising with other moms is a great way to meet other babies. They'll be your child's friends in the future, but right now they are there simply to highlight the beauteousness of your progeny—something that, good friend that you are, you'll keep entirely to yourself.

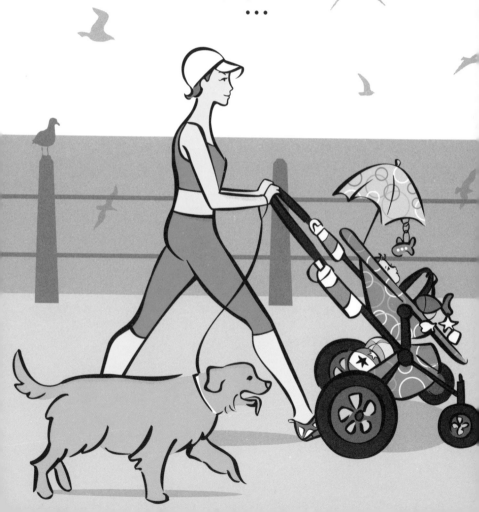

CHAPTER 5

BEYOND SIX MONTHS

Staying on track

. . .

You made it—six whole months. It's quite a milestone. And what a half-year it's been. Let's review: you had a baby; you struggled with and mastered all those deceptively simple (but staggeringly complicated) baby care skills like breast-feeding, diapering, and packing a diaper bag that weighs less than twenty pounds; you nurtured a baby that sleeps (some of the time), eats, laughs, plays, gurgles, snuggles, and maybe even sits up by himself; and along with all that, you actually found time to exercise. Yup, you're pretty spectacular.

Now that you've strengthened and toned your various key muscle groups, it's time to introduce more cardiovascular elements into your workout regime, beyond your daily walk. In this chapter, we talk in more depth about all the different forms of aerobic exercise that you (and your baby) can try, both with and without equipment. And we also discuss the incredible benefits of yoga for postpartum women.

And because your life will, inevitably, start to get busier from now on—your baby's bigger and more mobile; you may have returned to full- or part-time work; you're grappling with people's (erroneous) perception that the nesting and nurturing phase is well and truly over now that your baby is no longer a tiny newborn—there are also some hints and tips for staying on track and sticking with the program. For while you may feel like a relatively old hand at this mom thing, remember that you still have years and years ahead of you to be a fit mama.

• • •

1. GET ON YOUR BIKE

Cardio workouts with equipment

• • •

Cardiovascular ("cardio") or aerobic exercise is, as we've said, any activity that gets your heart working a little faster and increases your breathing rate. If you can get your cardio fix from the kind of activity that fits in with your daily life—walking to the store, going on a weekend hike—that's great. But if your lifestyle doesn't facilitate these kinds of fitness opportunities, then think about investing in the kind of in-home equipment that makes breaking a sweat a little easier. And there's one big advantage to in-home exercise equipment—it makes it very easy to exercise and keep an eye on your baby at the same time.

Cardio equipment runs the gamut from cheap to expensive. You can spend a few dollars on a jump rope or a few thousand on an elliptical trainer. We'll discuss the pros and cons of each, and then you'll be in a better position to make the right fiscal call.

Expensive stuff.
• • • • • • •

Bicycle. You have two ways to go—stationary or traditional. Either way, cycling is great aerobic exercise. If you're old-school and hanker to reclaim the ten-speed that's languishing in your garage, know that your baby will have to stay home while you enjoy the wind on your face. And there are a couple of other things to consider. If you haven't ridden a bike since fifth grade, take it slowly. Also, using the road as a cyclist is a whole different matter than driving in a car. It can be an eye-opening experience, so keep your wits about you, and wear the appropriate protective clothing, especially a helmet.

If you're looking for cardiovascular exercise that you can do with your baby in sight, a stationary bicycle might be right up your alley. A recumbent one is better if you

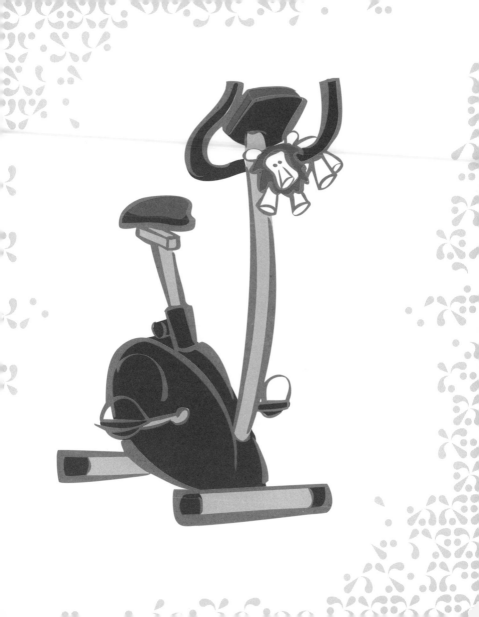

have some lower back pain. Make sure you are fully healed before you commit to spending time on the saddle (you know what we're saying). And be cognizant of safety—some models have useful safety features like a chain guard and spokes that aren't exposed to small fingers, which is vital if you plan on exercising near your child. And why wouldn't you? The sight of you exerting yourself, red in the face, and poised on a strange contraption could keep your baby amused for hours.

Elliptical trainer. It walks! It runs! It climbs! And so do you. An elliptical trainer can be a great lower body workout, and models that include handlebars that move as you do offer an upper body workout too. The downside? They're big and they're expensive, especially if you want all the bells and whistles. Be sure that you have space for one in your house, and make sure it's in a well-ventilated room where there's a place for your baby to sit in her car seat or bouncy chair. You may be tempted to situate it in the living room to watch TV as you exercise: be sure that your slightly oversensitive postpartum aesthetic sense can cope with all that metal and pleather amid your charmingly decorated home. (Although, on second thought, it's not a bad way to get used to the avalanche of unsightly plastic that will invade your adult environment over the years to come.)

Stair stepper. As with an elliptical trainer, it's most beneficial if used on a regular basis—a few minutes every day is always better and safer than a massive blowout on weekends. It's also fun to monitor your heart rate and see how many calories you're burning, but be sure to listen to your body first and foremost, rather than simply focusing on the LCD dial in front of you. Setting goals for yourself is fine, but let your body have the final word. Stair steppers let you decide on the level of your workout, so you can increase the intensity as you get fitter and braver. Be careful to use the handrails only to support yourself—leaning on them promotes poor posture and, in any case, means that your workout isn't as effective.

In general, if you're intent on buying a serious piece of equipment, take a good look around to find the safest and most child-friendly one. Moving parts can get hot, and there are plenty of places for small fingers to get trapped. Equipment like this is made for adults, so the level of "childproofing" is something that you may have to assess for yourself.

While this type of equipment—stationary cycles, elliptical trainers, stair steppers, and good old-fashioned treadmills, for that matter—may cost big bucks, they have one big built-in advantage. The money you spend on them may serve as an incentive to use them on a regular basis, say, every day for fifteen minutes, increasing time and frequency as your levels of fitness and stamina increase. Plus, they're so big you can't really ignore the fact that you bought it and now you have to use it.

Equipment that's less expensive is, by definition, more low commitment and may rely more on your innate desire to get fit in order to get used consistently. If this varies on a minute-by-minute basis, think carefully about how you spend your money. (Physical therapy balls, once deflated, fit quite inconspicuously at the back of your closet.)

Cheap stuff.
• • • •

Aerobic step. This is literally the step you use in a step class. Even if you haven't encountered one in person, you'll no doubt have seen one in action on an infomercial. They're not super-expensive and are easily available in most sports stores or online. Don't think about trying to adapt something you already have at home—a rickety old bench or the step stool you use to get the turkey platter off the high shelf once a year, for example. Proper aerobic steps are designed to sit firmly on the ground and absorb impact in a nonjarring way.

Jump rope. With a little space and a little stamina, a jump rope is a great exercise tool. Wear good-fitting exercise shoes, and pick your jumping surface carefully—choose one that limits friction. (Your downstairs neighbors really don't want to hear your sneakers squeaking on your hardwood living room floor all afternoon.) Make soft, little jumps, and land on the balls of your feet—go for minimal impact, and be kind to your joints. Remember, your goal isn't to leap as high as possible; you're jumping over a very thin rope, not a fifteen-foot boa constrictor.

Physical therapy ball. This is a wonderful and versatile piece of equipment. It's fun to sit on with your baby, and it can be the focus of some really great exercises. Plus, you may already have one at home, as a small memento of the hours you spent in labor.

Mini-trampoline. Aficionados tout a number of impressive health benefits that can be derived from use of this relatively inexpensive piece of equipment. Regular rebounding, as it's called, is said to improve the circulation of your lymphatic system (which helps eliminate toxins from your body), improve bone density and muscular strength (because of the gravitational pull that your body experiences when rebounding), and, like all cardiovascular exercises, strengthen your heart and lungs.

The following exercise circuit makes use of the less expensive pieces of cardio-focused equipment that we discussed above. (If you don't have all of them, simply adjust the circuit accordingly.) Best of all, you can do it at home. It's the kind of routine that may require some motivation—after all, the lure of the sofa may prove greater than the thought of running up and down stairs a few times. But on the plus side, it's cheap, it's effective, and it's a great way to keep your child entertained, as you can move him from room to room as you switch from one piece of equipment to the next or just wave at him as you flash by.

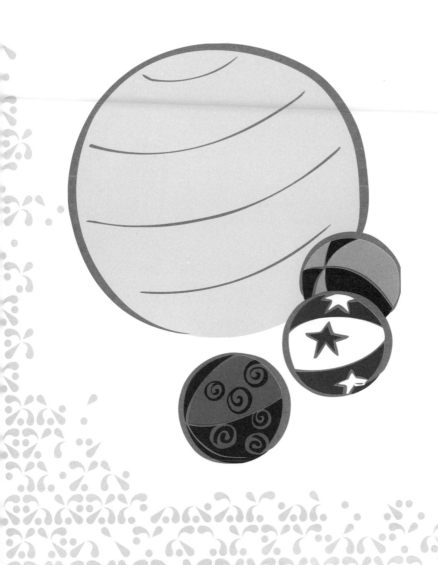

EXERCISE: YOUR IN-HOME CARDIO CIRCUIT

Frequency: Two circuits, twice a day

As always, be sure to stretch well before you begin (and when you're done, too). Music may help you feel more motivated and make your workout more fun.

Part 1: Step It Up!

Equipment: The stairs in your home or, preferably, an aerobic step

Start by mastering the rhythm—up with your left foot, up with your right foot, back down with your left foot, back down with your right foot, and so on. Try to maintain a regular, sprightly pace for at least sixty seconds.

Part 2: Jump That Rope!

Equipment: A jump rope—it should be long enough for you to step on the middle and still hold each end at midchest

Set yourself an attainable target, according to your stamina and sure-footedness—something like twenty consecutive jumps without stumbling. Or decide to jump for thirty seconds. But listen to your body: jumping rope can be surprisingly tiring, so if you feel fatigued, reassess your target number of jumps.

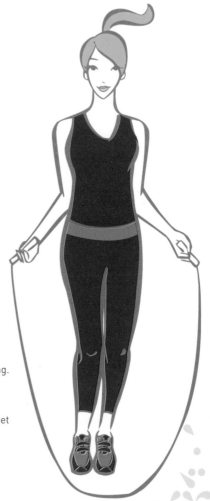

Part 3: Push It Up!

Equipment: A physical therapy ball

1   Lie across the ball on your tummy, and roll forward, carrying your body's weight on your hands until the ball is under your lower legs.

2   Bend at the elbows, and lower your body toward the floor.

3   Keep your body as straight as you can, all the way from your shoulders to your toes, as you return to your starting position.

4   Repeat ten times.

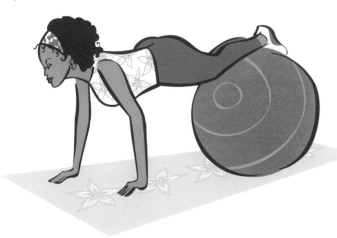

Part 4: Get Rebounding!

Equipment: A mini-trampoline or rebounder

If you're new to rebounding, learn to bounce while your (bare) feet remain in contact with the mat. Start with a five-minute session, and increase the time you spend bouncing when you feel more confident.

2. AND THEN GET OFF IT

Cardio workouts without equipment

• • •

Having discussed cardiovascular exercise that relies on your willingness to spend at least a few dollars on some equipment, it's time to get back to basics. Some of the most beneficial forms of exercise require nothing more than a decent pair of sneakers and an appreciation of the great outdoors or a public swimming pool within striking distance.

Walking.
• • • • • •

We've touted the benefits elsewhere in this book, so it suffices to say that brisk walking is fantastic aerobic exercise that your stroller-bound baby will enjoy too. But make sure that your walk is brisk, and be careful not to slump over the handlebars.

Running.
• • • • • •

If you ran halfway seriously before you got pregnant (or even during your pregnancy), this is something that you can pick up with relative ease postpartum. You know your old body, and you probably have a good feel for your new body. If you're new to running but feel like trying it out, then go for it—while following these guidelines, of course.

Get fitted for good running shoes. Go to a reputable sports store, and spend the money that you saved on your rebounder, resistance bands, and physical therapy ball on some top-notch athletic shoes.

Wear a supportive bra. And breast-feed your baby before running, for maximum boob comfort.

Choose your route with care. Remember to turn around and head for home when you're halfway tired, so you won't need to call for emergency backup (i.e., a friend with a car).

Run with a jogging stroller. Wide wheels and a well-sprung chassis make it a more comfortable ride for your child. Don't try running with your everyday umbrella stroller—it's simply not as maneuverable.

Watch your joints. Running, or even a slow jog, creates impact. Take it slowly, and if it hurts, stop.

Don't leave home without your well-toned pelvic floor muscles. Even so, you may find that running causes *stress incontinence*—the leaking of a little pee. Take this as a gentle reminder that you need to keep up with your Kegel exercises.

Mix it up. Interspersing a couple of minutes of running with a couple of minutes of brisk walking is a great way to feel the benefits of powerful cardiovascular exercise, while lessening the impact on your joints.

Swimming.

There's probably no better aerobic exercise than swimming. The water supports your body and virtually eliminates the risk of injury to your muscles and joints. As well as improving your cardiovascular capacity, regular swimming will help develop your muscular strength, your stamina, and your flexibility. Exercising in water keeps the body comfortably cool, and swimming laps can be very mentally therapeutic— the monotony gives you focused space in which to ponder deeper issues, and as this is something that requires the participation of a babysitter, it's great *you* time.

But if swimming laps isn't quite your thing, know that it isn't the only way you can benefit from aquatic exercise. Consider joining an aquatic aerobics class—your local sports center may well have classes specifically for postpartum women—or head to your local pool, and try this little routine that'll give you a full-body aquatic workout.

EXERCISE: WATER WORKS

The water's resistance makes these easy exercises highly effective, and in fact, you could end up burning up to 700 calories per hour of aquatic aerobic activity. Wear aqua shoes if you like: they'll give you more traction on the pool floor. And remember that you can still get dehydrated even when you're surrounded by gallons of water. Drink plenty before you head to the pool.

Part 1: Walking

To warm up, walk up and down the pool for five minutes.

Part 2: Jogging

Jog one or two lengths of the pool. (If you get tired, we'll let you walk part of the way.)

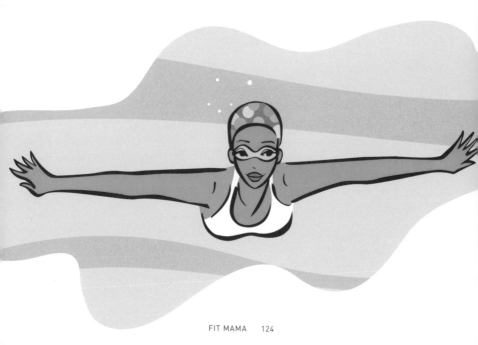

Part 3: Kicking

1   Hold on to the side of the pool (or grab a kickboard if you feel like moving around).

2   Allow your body to float up into a horizontal position, and start kicking with a swift but regular scissoring motion. Do two minutes—your hips, buttocks, and even your abdominals will thank you.

Part 4: Skiing

This is more your cross-country mode than your Olympic downhill or slalom. The important thing is to keep your arms and legs straight and move them back and forth as you make your way up and down the pool. Try to do two laps.

Part 5: Bouncing

Bouncing in water is a little like bouncing on a mini-trampoline. And it's certainly a lot better for you (and your joints) than jumping up and down on a hard, unresisting surface. Try to bounce for two minutes.

Part 6: Crunching

1   Stand with your back at the edge of the pool. Pull your elbows up onto the pool side.

2   Keep your legs straight, and bring them up slowly to make a 90-degree angle with your body. Hold this position for five seconds, keeping your breathing slow and steady. Lower your legs.

3   Repeat five times.

Part 7: Leg Lifting

1   Give your hips and buttocks a workout by holding onto the edge of the pool as you slowly bring your left leg up and out to the side. Bring it as high as you can go without rotating your ankle.

2   Repeat with your right leg. Do five sets of each.

Part 8: Squatting

This is great for your thighs and buttocks. With your feet apart, bend your knees, and "sit down" until your knees are behind your toes. Stand up tall. Repeat five to ten times.

Aqua aerobics is a great way to enjoy the benefits of exercising in water if you aren't a strong swimmer. But if you aren't a strong swimmer, don't go into the pool alone; cajole a friend to come and join you. This may also increase your comfort level if you're a bit self-conscious about the impression you're creating as you jump up and squat low while those hard-core lap swimmers zoom by you.

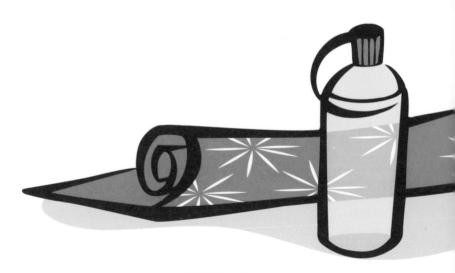

3. AND THEN TAKE A DEEP BREATH

Workouts without the cardio

• • •

After all that strengthening and aerobicizing, you may have a yen for something a little less active, a little more relaxing. Good news—you've come to the right place. Welcome to yoga.

The benefits of yoga.
• • •

For something so outwardly gentle and measured, yoga really packs a punch in terms of health benefits, both physical and mental. It improves your circulatory system and cardiovascular efficiency; it enhances your strength, flexibility, and muscle tone; and it raises your energy levels and make you feel less fatigued. You can look forward to a better posture. You'll feel more supple. And it can even lower your blood pressure.

Yoga classes, even ones specifically for postpartum women, are relatively easy to find. And they can be great. You get instruction, group support, and a nice environment in which you and your baby can hang out and bond over (or under) poses with fabulous names. But if you can't get out to a class, yoga is one of the easiest exercise disciplines you can do at home. Just invest in a decent yoga mat (for your comfort and safety), and you're good to go.

Start with the following sequence of six different yoga poses (a couple of which actually incorporate your baby into the action). You can pick and choose the ones you like best—the ones that seem to best ease any particular areas of discomfort— or, for maximum effect, work on accomplishing the sequence as a whole. But take your time. There's no hurry either to master the poses or to complete the sequence. It's more important that you feel comfortable doing the poses and concentrate on breathing slowly, steadily, and deeply throughout, in order to promote real relaxation.

YOGA POSE #1: BOUND ANGLE POSE (BADDHA KONASANA)

Want flexibility in the hips and groin? This one is for you.

1   Sit flat on the mat with a blanket under your buttocks for support.

2   Bend your legs, open your knees, and put the soles of your feet together.

3   Bring your heels close to your pubic bone.

4   Be sure that you can feel each buttock firmly on the support as you lift up the sides of your body.

5   Widen your collarbones, and push your shoulder blades backward.

6   Stretch from your inner groin to the knee (rather than forcing your legs down to the ground).

7   Concentrate on your breathing as you hold the pose.

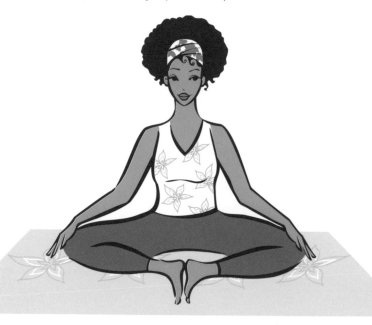

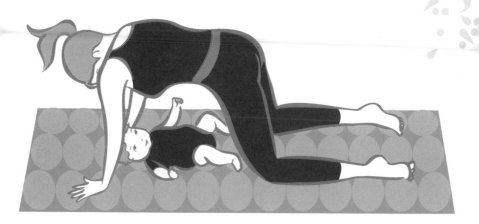

YOGA POSE #2: CAT POSE (MARJARYASANA)

This simple, baby-friendly pose is great for relieving lower backache, strengthening your abdominal muscles, and creating flexibility in your spine.

1   Place your baby on his back, just underneath your arms so that he's looking up at you.

2   Move onto your hands and knees.

3   Inhale, look up, and arch your back slightly.

4   Exhale, round your back, and look down at your baby.

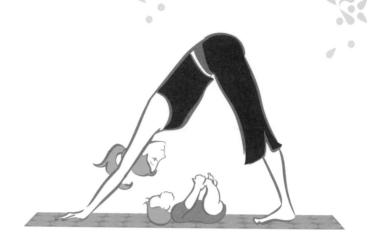

YOGA POSE #3: DOWNWARD-FACING DOG (ADHO MUKHA SVANASANA)
This pose stretches the spine and strengthens the legs. Again, it's one that your baby will enjoy participating in.

1 Lie your baby on her back on the mat, either in front of you or below you.

2 Start in a kneeling position, with your back to a wall.

3 Turn your toes under, and lift your sitting bones high up to the ceiling, internally rotating the tops of your thighs.

4 Press the backs of your hamstrings toward the wall behind you.

5 Press your hands firmly into the floor, and extend your arms.

YOGA POSE #4: UPWARD-FACING DOG (URDHVA MUKHA SVANASANA)

This pose helps relieve stiff shoulders and upper and lower back tension. It also opens the chest, which can help relieve depression.

1   Lie facedown, with your feet hip-width apart and your legs active. (You should be able to rotate your legs at the hip.)

2   Place your hands on the mat, just below your shoulders.

3   Press your hands into the mat, and leading with your sternum, bring your upper torso off the mat and your pelvis closer to your hands.

4   Hold this pose for a few seconds (or longer if you can) as you concentrate on your breathing.

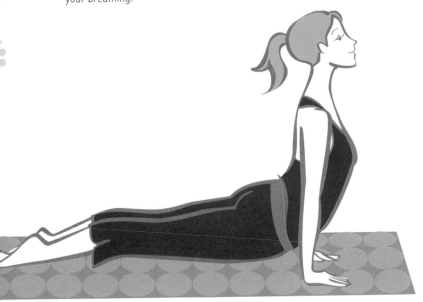

YOGA POSE #5: CHILD'S POSE (BALASANA)

This pose gently stretches the lower back, lengthens the spine, and releases tension in your back and neck. It's very calming and can actually help lower blood pressure.

1 Kneel on the floor.

2 Open your knees slightly, and bring your big toes together.

3 Bend your body forward until your forehead touches the floor.

4 Hold this pose for a few minutes, and let your mind and body relax.

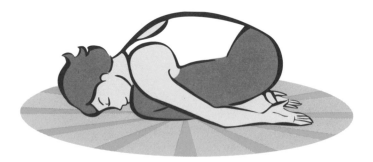

YOGA POSE #6: RECLINING BOUND ANGLE POSE
(SUPTA BADDHA KONASANA)

This relaxing, rejuvenating, and stress-relieving pose is great for new mothers. Using a bolster supports the body and allows the chest to open (which you'll appreciate, seeing as you spend way too much time hunching your shoulders over a variety of baby-related tasks). It also takes pressure off the pelvic area, opens the hips and groin, and encourages blood flow into those areas, which can alleviate backache. This pose is a great one to end on. See if you can hold it for ten minutes or more.

1   Place a bolster behind you with a folded blanket on it to support your head and neck.

2   Sit in front of it with your sacrum—the very lowest part of your spine—touching the bolster.

3   Put the soles of your feet together, allowing your knees to fall to the sides.

4   Lie back on the bolster so that your buttocks and legs are on the floor. Your torso should be supported by the bolster, with your head and neck supported by the blanket.

5   Take your arms out to the sides of your body, palms facing upward.

6   Breathe as you hold the pose.

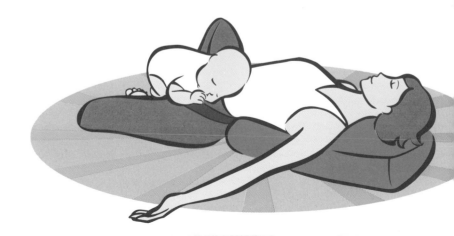

4. BECAUSE YOU LAUGHED IN THE FACE OF MORNING SICKNESS

How you know you can stick with the program

• • •

Your baby is turning out to be a very busy young person. There's a lot of playing, a lot of eating, some sleeping, and a lot of being demanding. When you factor in all the other jobs you have to do—the one that pays you a salary and the ones that don't—you may find that there's not a lot of time, or energy, left over for a fitness routine.

But please don't doubt your ability to stay the distance. Never fear that you'll never be a fit mama. The going may be tough at times, but we have complete faith in you. Why, don't you know that you have the endurance of a long-distance runner and twice the willpower? Here's how we know that you can do it.

- **Because you grew a baby.** You were strong and patient for some forty weeks. You lived an abstemious and virtuous life. You denied yourself alcohol, eschewed late nights, and opted for low-heeled shoes (even though they make your ankles look thick). If you can do that, you can do anything.

- **Because you gave birth to a baby.** Delivering a baby is probably the most arduous and intense thing you'll ever do. (Until you do it again, of course.) What's that compared to a bit of exercise-induced sweating?

- **Because you choose cottage cheese as well as ice cream.** You've got a very good sense of how to treat your body right. At mealtimes, particularly, your sense of self-preservation kicks in. You know that to do every thing you do *and* exercise consistently on top of it all you have to put the right kind of fuel into your body. But you also know how motivating the occasional reward can be. Congratulations on seeking—and finding—a modicum of balance in your busy life.

- **Because you've perfected the art of the power nap.** You've gotten really good at making do with less sleep, with fewer manicures and hair appointments, and with no space in the bathroom cabinet. (Those economy-size boxes of baby wipes sure do take up a lot of room.) Similarly, you're an expert at finding little corners of your day for a quick yoga pose or two, converting a stroll to the grocery store into a power walk, and inspiring your significant other to babysit while you swim a few laps at the local pool.

- **Because you can calm a cranky baby with no toys.** You're a resourceful young woman. You can keep your baby highly entertained just by blowing raspberries on his tummy; you can whip up a satisfactory supper from the contents of your refrigerator *five whole days after your last trip to the grocery store*; and you can find an opportunity to exercise in your own home, on a rainy day, and with only a physical therapy ball for company.

- **Because you laughed in the face of morning sickness.** You knew that your green complexion and the swells of nausea that punctuated the first trimester or two were all for a good cause. Just like you know that exercising, while it may not fit entirely conveniently into your new schedule, or your new state of mind, really is worth it in the long run.

CHAPTER 6
HEY, FIT MAMA
You go, girl!

• • •

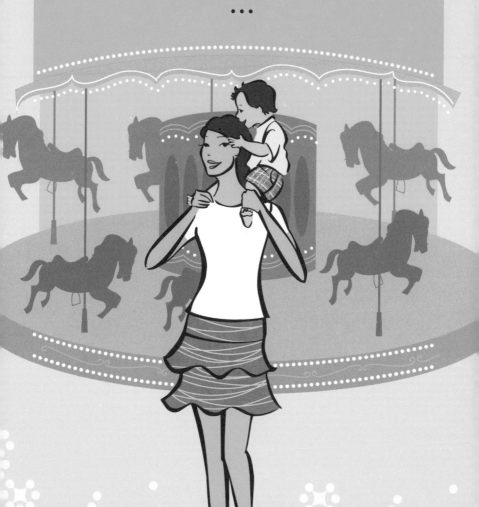

It's official. You're a fit mama. It's been at least a year since the birth of your baby and months since you made the commitment to make exercise a regular part of your life. Your pelvic floor and abdominal muscles have been well and truly tightened (no more inadvertent peeing for you); your posture is in fine form; you've introduced elements of strength training and cardiovascular exercise into your routine; and you're an old hand at a yoga pose or two. Your head's in a great place, and your body looks even better. You've made amazing progress, and we're proud of you.

But (and wouldn't you just know it?) it's right about now that the hard work really starts. This is when you have to dig deep into your reserves of willpower and endurance and make a firm and solemn vow to stay on the path that you've so ably forged. Because, having scaled the mountain of physical fitness, there's a teeny-weeny chance that you might start to relax your efforts. There's the real possibility that your exercise routine might become a little predictable—a little dull, even. For one reason or another, you might simply decide to rest on your laurels (a.k.a. the sofa). All of which means that you need to keep your exercise routine fresh, exciting, and above all, motivating.

In this chapter, we'll explore some strategies that can help you revamp your workout and keep you focused. And because your life is getting busier as your baby gets older, we have some thoughts on how you can find balance in your life as you struggle with the competing demands of being a mom, holding down a job, keeping your family happy, and being a partner. And just to throw a curveball into your otherwise calm and easy life (relatively speaking), we'll discuss how you can successfully manage a second pregnancy along with being a fit mama. And if you can do *that*, you can do anything!

• • •

1. ARE WE THERE YET?

Learning when you're finally post-postpartum

• • •

Thumbing through your dictionary for the definition of *postpartum,* you might turn up something vague and unhelpful like "the period following birth." Check with one of your pregnancy or baby care books, and you might find an answer that's slightly more long-winded, perhaps something like "the postpartum period is the first year after the birth of your child." Of course, neither definition is any use to anyone who's looking for an answer as to when they might confidently expect *not* to be postpartum anymore. And, in any case, can you really expect to be free of the physical and emotional effects of pregnancy, labor, delivery, and the first year of child rearing the minute your child turns one?

The short answer to questions like *when can I expect my body to function the same way it functioned before I gave birth?* and, more important, *when can I expect my tummy to return to its former six-pack (or, at least, two-pack) sleekness?* is that having a baby has some effects that don't magically disappear after a conveniently prearranged period of time. Few women walk out the other side looking like they've spent a couple of weeks relaxing on a beach in Maui. Your body, as we've discussed, may never be the same again. And as for your head—who knew that you'd spend hours in fascinated conversation about breast infections or analyzing the color and consistency of your young one's poop? So, in a sense, once you've had a baby, you're postpartum forever. If that's an option too scary to contemplate, simply pick your personal favorite from the list of postpartum definitions that follow.

You stop being postpartum . . .
. . . . . .

. . . one year after your baby's birth. While this is the most popular definition, remember that different women recover from pregnancy and childbirth at different speeds. One year on, and you may feel in better physical shape than you did before you had your baby. Or you may not. But be warned—setting yourself that one-year deadline may cause you unnecessary anxiety about your performance if you still lack the energy required to get you and your eleven-month-old out of your respective jammies before noon.

. . . when you stop breast-feeding. While the American Academy of Pediatrics recommends "exclusive breast-feeding for approximately the first six months and support for breast-feeding for the first year and beyond as long as mutually desired by mother and child" (February 2005), your personal circumstances and preferences may dictate otherwise. Your child may self-wean sooner that you wanted; you may have to stop nursing because you're on medication that's incompatible with breast-feeding; you may choose to nurse your child well into his second or third year; or you may get pregnant again before you stop breast-feeding your firstborn. You may consider yourself no longer postpartum when you stop breast-feeding, but clearly, that's a time frame that varies from mom to mom.

. . . when you become pregnant again. Of course, not all mothers go on to have subsequent children, but for the sake of argument, let's say that eighteen months after the birth of your first child, you become pregnant again. Does your new pregnancy signal the end of your postpartum period? Or is it, in fact, entirely possible to be both pregnant and postpartum at the same time? Or (more likely) are you simply too exhausted to even care, as you battle a fractious toddler alongside hormonal mood swings and nausea?

. . . when you want to be. The truth is, while we'd love to give the post-partum period a tidy time line, it's just not that easy. You'll always be different after you've had a baby, physically and emotionally. The trick is not to let being post-partum (in the broadest sense of the word) define who you are or dictate what you can and can't do. You're a woman, first and foremost, and a mother, and therein lies your real power.

2. KICKING IT UP A NOTCH

How to advance your fitness routine

• • •

By now, you've probably reached a satisfying comfort level with your exercise program. That's both a good and a bad thing. On the one hand, when exercise becomes as natural as breathing, when you feel bereft if you have to miss a session, it's clear that you've integrated fitness well and truly into your life. But on the other, when your routine becomes too easy, too comfortable, too *boring*, then it's time to change things up. Here are our suggestions for putting a different spin on your workout.

Try something new.

If you're getting stuck in a rut, revisit the earlier chapters of this book. Maybe aqua aerobics didn't appeal too much three months ago, but heck, now that the weather's warmer, what could be nicer than a trip to the outdoor pool? And now that you have more confidence in your physical abilities—and the fear that you'll be the straggler in the group starts to recede—maybe this is a good time to hook up with your mom friends for one of those gnarly hiking-up-a-large-hill-with-a-heavy-stroller afternoons.

Go to a class.

If your fifteen laps a day three times a week and thirty minutes of yoga every other day makes you yawn, think about trying some group exercise. By now, you can consider classes not labeled "postpartum," so seize the opportunity to venture into unknown territory. Ever fancied kickboxing? It's a great workout and lots of fun too. Or how about dance? Dance schools offer classes for all abilities, so never fear that you'll be the only klutz in the studio. The important thing is to keep your workout varied so that you stay interested.

Work out on your own.
· · · · · · · · ·

It's great that you've joined classes—as we've said more than once, working out with a group can be both fun and inspiring. But now that you're a bit of an expert, consider the possibility that your class simply isn't pushing you hard enough. This might be a good time to go solo for a few of your weekly exercise sessions. You may find motivation easier to come by when you're trying to best the time you made on your last run, rather than chatting with your neighbor in your yoga class.

And, if you'd like to introduce some new elements into your at-home exercise program, consider the following exercises. They target the areas that new moms tend to complain about most—the hips and thighs. And as a bonus to the economy conscious, they also make use of some of the equipment that you invested in a few months ago.

EXERCISE: THE BIG SQUEEZE
Frequency: Twice a day

You'll need your physical therapy ball for this one.

1 Lie on your back on a mat.

2 Hold the physical therapy ball between your lower legs and ankles.

3 Raise the ball into the air as you apply pressure to the sides of the ball. Your legs should create about a 45-degree angle with the floor.

4 Hold this position as you breathe slowly in and out twice.

5 Lower the ball to the floor, and breathe.

6 Repeat ten times.

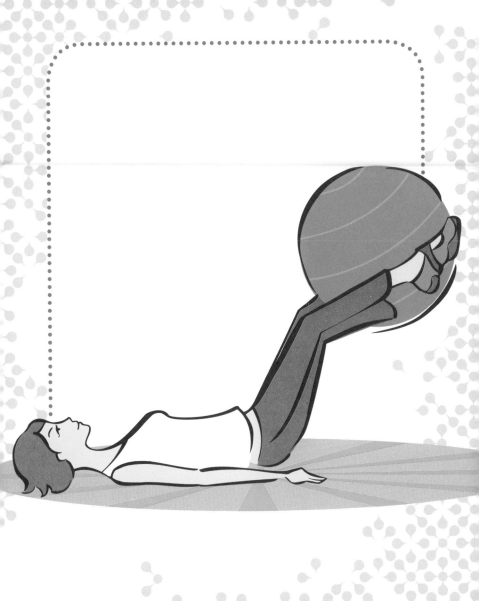

EXERCISE: STRETCH IT OUT

Frequency: Twice a day

Get out your resistance band for this great exercise that'll work your hips and inner thighs.

1   With feet hip-width apart, stand on your resistance band.

2   Grasp the ends of the band in both hands.

3   Slowly lean to your left while stretching your right leg out to the side. You should feel resistance from the band on the outside edge of your right foot.

4   Return your body to the starting position, and repeat.

5   Do ten on each side of your body.

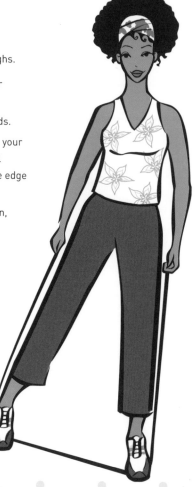

EXERCISE: LEG LIFTS
Frequency: Twice a day

This is a very simple exercise that, done right, can be highly effective in firming up those troublesome thigh and buttock muscles.

1   Lie on the left side of your body. Keep your body straight, with your knees and toes pointing forward. Rest your head on your left arm.

2   Raise your upper leg so that it makes an angle of about 45 degrees (or less, if that's more comfortable for you).

3   With this angle as your starting position, slowly lower and raise your leg a few inches with a controlled, regular motion. You should feel the stretch in your outer thigh and buttocks.

4   Do one set of ten, and then repeat with your other leg.

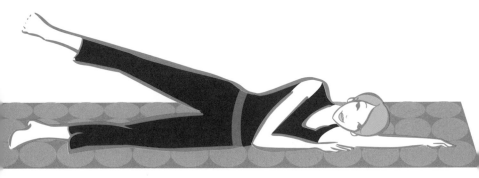

3. WHATEVER DID I DO BEFORE I HAD A BABY?

Finding the time to find the balance

• • •

Everything gets a whole lot busier once you throw a baby into the mix. Not to mention the fact that you (yes, *you*) have made the significant commitment to make exercise an important part of your week (if not your day) for a whole slew of very good reasons. Right about now, you may be wondering how you can possibly fit it all in. We're not going to lie to you—it's not easy. Your obligations have increased exponentially, and you still have all the old stuff going on (relationships, work, family, home, money) to boot.

But what comes first? What takes priority? The short answer is *you*. Because, if you meet your own needs, you'll be in a much better place to meet everybody else's needs. As you're on page 146, it's fairly apparent that exercise is one of your needs—it keeps you healthy, it keeps you sane, and it helps you be the energetic and motivated person that you want to be (and have to be, considering how full your life is). But the big question remains—how do you find the time to fit exercise in? Consider the following strategies.

Squeeze more time out of the day.
• • • • • • • • • •

True, there are only a certain number of hours in the day, but it's possible to make more of the ones that you have. Go to bed half an hour earlier, and right there you've found time for an invigorating thirty-minute, early morning run before the rest of your house stirs. Give up a couple of your weekly television shows (hard, we know, but you'll find it liberating once you get over the withdrawal symptoms). Limit your gossipy phone calls to just one or two evenings a week (and think of the money you'll save on your long-distance bill).

Simplify your life.

Make detailed shopping lists so that you can be in and out of the grocery store in a fraction of the time. If you're fixing dinner, double the quantity and freeze half. Don't fret about eating from the microwave. Stop buying clothes that need ironing (or stop caring about those unnoticeable wrinkles). OK, so maybe we're starting to sound like one of those yes-you-can-be-superwoman magazine articles (for which we apologize), but we have your best interests at heart, and anything that simplifies domestic chores can only mean more personal time for you and your workout.

Multitask before you get to the office.

Write a report or read a strategy document during your commute (that's got to be at least an extra hour a day you've just found for yourself), and promise that you'll never bring work home (unless your job depends on it).

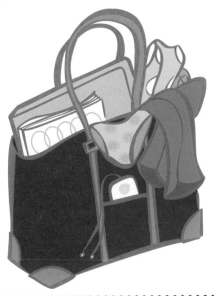

Work out at work.

······

If you're the kind of person who diligently sits at her desk through lunch, have a word with yourself. You need to take a break at some point during the day. (This is especially true if you've sacrificed your trashy-magazine-reading morning commute in favor of work-related activities.) If you are lucky enough to be within striking distance of a gym, it's entirely possible to get a decent workout in a lunch hour (fifteen minutes to get there and change; twenty-five minutes on the elliptical trainer and treadmill or in the pool; twenty minutes showering and striding back to the office). It sounds like a mission, but as you know, exercise is very invigorating, and you'll probably find that your typical midafternoon sleepy slump becomes a thing of the past. (Bring your lunch from home, and you won't even need to schedule time to spend the best part of $10 on something disappointing with *panini* in its name.)

Keep working out with your baby.

··········

Maybe your twelve- or eighteen-month-old is a little too big for the front pack or wreaks havoc at your peaceful mom-and-baby yoga class, but there are plenty of other ways you and your child can enjoy each other's company while you get some exercise. Consider joining a baby gym class—while ostensibly intended for your young friend, there's no reason why you can't do some stretches and sit-ups while your baby is rolling around on the big, squishy mat. Walk everywhere you can—make the weekend trip to the store your exercise for the day by walking there and back and buying some really heavy things so you increase the resistance for the journey home. Take your toddler to any wide open space—the park, the beach, even the mall—and you'll burn an incredible number of calories just keeping up with him.

Exercise little and often.

··········

In an ideal world, you'd have the luxury (and the time) to exercise for about forty-five minutes a day, three, four, or even five days a week. But *we* don't live in an ideal world, and we're presuming that *you* don't either. That being said, it's perfectly acceptable to break up that forty-five minute workout into three more manageable fifteen-minute chunks—say, some pre-breakfast yoga, a brisk walk in your lunch hour, and an evening run.

Streamline your workout.

There's no reason you have to keep your strength training and cardio workouts separate, and in fact, mixing them into the same session means you'll get the benefits of both in half the time. Alternate a few minutes of cardio exercise with a few minutes of strength training, and you'll burn fat and build muscle at the same time.

Think of your family.

Share the wealth, and spread the fun. Drag your partner to the park or the beach, and throw a Frisbee around. This is a great spectator sport for a baby.

If fitting exercise into your life like this sounds horribly frantic, that's because it is. Nobody ever had a baby because it would make their lives more convenient and less stressful. Children take up a lot of room and take a lot from you. They give it back, in spades, but it's always going to be a balancing act, and to be honest, it never really changes. Sure, you may look forward to the day when your baby isn't nursing through the night or lurching from one set of sniffles to the next, but there's always *something* to contend with (homework, after-school activities, birthday parties, and first dates are just some of the issues you'll encounter before too long). Start putting yourself and your exercise routine first, and you'll be making a commitment that's going to benefit you—for the rest of your life.

4. THE ULTIMATE DEFINITION
OF MULTITASKING

Being postpartum, pregnant, and *staying fit*

• • •

Well, you did it (became a fit mama). And, oops, you did it again (became pregnant). But the latter state of affairs is no reason why you should forgo your obvious talent for the former.

Being prenatal and postpartum is a fairly special set of circumstances but one with which a commitment to exercise is entirely compatible. As we said way back in chapter 1, you're likely to have a healthier and more relaxed pregnancy if you exercise consistently and sensibly for the full forty weeks—although you may find it difficult to accept the few limitations that come with pregnancy (exercise maven that you now are).

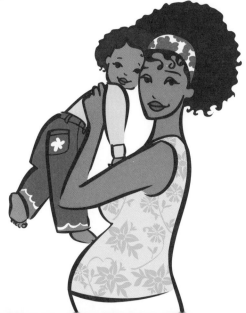

At this point, we're assuming that either you didn't exercise during your pregnancy the first time around or, more charitably, that so much has happened since then that the specifics of your very first prenatal workout are just a dim and distant memory. With that in mind, here are a few pointers to enjoying a successful prenatal/post-partum workout:

Tell your doctor that you're exercising.

Any information that's material to you and your pregnancy should always be shared with your practitioner. Of course, feel free to mention that you're a bit of an expert on the exercise front.

Listen to your body.

Be particularly aware of signs that it's time to stop, such as feeling faint or short of breath. If you experience any vaginal bleeding or contractions, contact your doctor or midwife as soon as possible.

Stay off your back.

After the first trimester, avoid exercises that require you to lie on your back, as the weight of the uterus can put pressure on the inferior vena cava (a pretty major vein). This can make you dizzy and reduce the blood supply to your brain and to your baby.

Exercise some caution.

For the postpartum woman, few activities are out of bounds. Pregnancy imposes more restraints, especially where the risk of falling or serious injury is greater. You probably shouldn't indulge in horseback riding, downhill skiing, and contact sports.

Do what you're good at.

Depending on your fitness level, this may not be the time to take up something new. Keep running, if that's what you've been doing. If it isn't, stick to swimming, yoga, or brisk walking.

Consider your body.

Now that you're pregnant again, your body may go into what we in the trade call *autopregnancy mode*, which means that you may get much bigger much faster than last time. Balance may become quite the problem rather quickly.

Think of your wibbly-wobbly joints.

Remember all that talk of the pregnancy hormone *relaxin*? We mentioned it in the context of safe postpartum exercise, but it's even more pertinent to safe prenatal exercise. Be kind to your joints, and avoid repeated jumping on hard surfaces.

Revisit your workout regularly.

Your body's changing all the time. And by *changing*, we mean *getting bigger*. The workout that worked well for you in months two and three may not be so much fun when you're seven or eight months pregnant.

Enroll in a class.

If you're not sure what's safe or what's important, enroll in classes specifically for pregnant women. Having confirmed the credentials and experience of your instructor, you can be sure that you're getting a workout that's both appropriate and beneficial.

Warm up, and stay cool.

Always remember to warm up well with some stretches before any exercise session, and avoid exercising outdoors in hot or humid weather (try to work out in a well-ventilated room if you can). And always, always drink water before, during, and after exercising.

Above all, have fun.

This is the perfect time, pregnant and postpartum as you are, to really enjoy all the physical and emotional benefits that regular exercise offers. But you don't need us to tell you that. After all, you're a fit mama now!

EPILOGUE

Fit mama, and beyond

• • •

Hurrah! You made it. Having gotten this far, it'd be a real shame not to maintain your current level of extraordinary and admirable fitness. But sticking with it can be one of the hardest fitness challenges you'll face in this whole amazing journey. With that in mind and by way of a few last nuggets of motivational advice, here is our top-ten list of reasons why you should definitely make a commitment to stay a fit mama.

10 Because you've learned to appreciate the beauty that's inherent in spandex.

9 Because you like having your butt where it is right now, as opposed to four inches lower.

8 Because keeping up with small children requires an incredible amount of stamina (and none of us is getting any younger).

7 Because you like how everybody tells you how good you look (even if you're vexed by how surprised they seem when they say it).

6 Because after growing a baby and giving birth, getting fit is the one thing that you've done that's all about you.

5 Because you confidently aspire to getting into your pre-pre-baby wardrobe.

4 Because one day you'll want your son's friends to have a bit of a crush on you.

3 Because you'll always need a cast-iron excuse for some regular alone time.

2 Because staying fit is still a reason to go shopping (even if you're only hanging out at sports stores).

And the number one reason:

1 Because you like how you feel—inside and out—when you're a fit mama.

INDEX